U.S. Fire Administration
Mission Statement

We provide National leadership to foster a solid foundation for our fire and emergency services stakeholders in prevention, preparedness, and response.

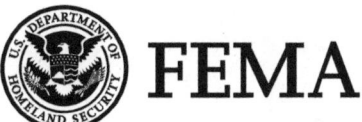 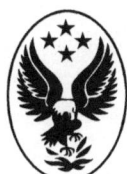

Developed for the U.S. Fire Administration (USFA) under Funding Opportunity Number DHS-10-USFA-105-000-04 by the National Emergency Medical Services Management Association.

Operational Templates and Guidance for EMS Mass Incident Deployment

This page was intentionally left blank.

Acknowledgements

The expert review panel for this publication was composed of senior Emergency Medical Service (EMS) leadership from a broad domain of stakeholders. Each contributed time and expertise to ensure that the final publication was useful to local level emergency planners in the EMS sector. Without their guidance and commitment to developing a practical, accurate, and relevant set of tools, this document would not have made it out of the planning stages. A special thank you goes out to Aarron Reinert, Steve Delahousey, and Mike McAdams for preparing and presenting information of key interest during the meeting for this project. Without the input and guidance from each stakeholder organization and their representatives on the expert review panel, this document would not have come to fruition.

Finally, Federal partners Rick Patrick and Bill Troup provided background and guidance as the project progressed from idea to implementation.

Expert Review Panel

National EMS Management Association: Project Team
Skip Kirkwood, NEMSMA President/Chief, Wake County EMS
Sean Caffrey, Project Manager/EMS Operations Program Manager, CDPHE
Jim Buell, Editor in Chief and Subject Matter Expert/Managing Partner, MTOG LLC
Keith Hart, Subject Matter Expert/Senior Partner, MTOG LLC
Bill Stanfield, Subject Matter Expert/Consultant, MTOG LLC
Rosalind Cooper, Editor, Wheat Ridge, Colorado
Jeff Dyar, Meeting Facilitator, The Far View Group, LLC

American Ambulance Association
Steve Delahousey, Vice President, American Medical Response

Center for Leadership Innovation and Research in EMS
Gary Wingrove, Director of Strategic Affairs, Mayo Medical Transport

International Association of EMS Chiefs
James Robinson, Operations Chief, Denver Health Paramedic Division

National Association of Emergency Medical Technicians
Don Lundy, EMS Director, Charleston County, South Carolina

International Association of Fire Chiefs
John Sinclair, Fire Chief/Emergency Manager, Kittitas Valley Fire Rescue

International Association of Fire Fighters
Lori Moore-Merrill, Assistant to the General President

International Association of Flight Paramedics
T.J. Kennedy, Program Manager/Assistant Vice President, Science Applications International Corporation (SAIC)

National Association of EMS Physicians
Dr. Kathy Rinnert, Director GEMSS/EMS Fellowship Programs, University of Texas Southwestern at Dallas
Dr. Brian Schwartz, Executive Lead, Sunnybrook-Osler Center for Prehospital Care

National Association of State EMS Officials
Joe Schmider, EMS Director, State of Pennsylvania

National Fire Protection Association
Ken Holland, Public Fire Protection Programs

National Highway Traffic Safety Administration
Gamunu "Gam" Wijetunge Office of Emergency Medical Services

National Volunteer Fire Council
Ken Knipper, Chair/EMS Rescue Section

Subject Matter Experts
Mike McAdams, Assistant Chief of Operations, Montgomery County Fire Rescue
Aarron Reinert, National EMS Advisory Committee, Executive Director, Lakes Region EMS
Al Martin, Fire Chief, City of Tuscaloosa, Alabama

U.S. Fire Administration
Bill Troup, Project Officer

United States Department of Health and Human Services
Jack Beall, Director, National Disaster Medical System

United States Department of Homeland Security
Rick Patrick, Director, Medical First Response Coordination, Office of Health Affairs
Dr. Michael Zanker, MD, Senior Medical Officer, Office of Health Affairs

Table of Contents

Introduction 1

SECTION I: Emergency Medical Services Deployment Templates 3
TEMPLATE 1: The Emergency Medical Services Emergency Operations Plan 3
TEMPLATE 2: Basic Hazard Vulnerability Analysis 6
TEMPLATE 3: Incident and Event Plans 9
TEMPLATE 4: Basic Incident Deployment Checklists 14

SECTION II: Mass Care Coordination Toolkit 19
Introduction to the Coordination Planning Toolkit 19
    High School Football Game 20
    Residential Medical Facility Evacuation 22
    County Fair 25
    Marathon or Similar Running Events 27
    Weather-Related Disaster Declaration 29
    Large College Sporting Event 31
    Political Assembly 34
    Auto Racing/Competition 36
    Cancer Walk 38

SECTION III: Case Studies in Mass Incident Deployment 41
Case 1: 2010 Bus Crash in Hartford, CT 41
Case 2: 2005 F3 Tornado in Marshall County, KY 43
Case 3: 2010 Veterans Administration Hospital Evacuation, Lebanon, PA 46
Case 4: 2008 Imperial Sugar Dixie Crystal Plant Fire, Port Wentworth, GA 49
Case 5: 2006 Woodward Dream Cruise, Berkley, MI 52
Case 6: 2010 Ironman Triathlon Event, St. George, UT 55
Case 7: 2004 Democratic National Convention, Boston, MA 57
Case 8: Annual Creation Music Festival, Mount Union, PA 60

SECTION IV: Policy Guidance for Mass Casualty Contingency Planning at Mass Gathering Events 63
Introduction 63
Relationship of Event Command to Responding Resources 67
Communications 68
Expanded Scope/Emerging Mass Casualty Incident Management Considerations 68
Mass Casualty Incident Planning Checklist 71
Incident Action Plan Safety and Risk Analysis, ICS Form 215A 73

SECTION V: Policy Guidance for Emergency Medical Services Aspects of Mass Shelter and Feeding 75
Emergency Medical Services Participation in Mass Shelter and Feeding 75
    Key Functional Roles and Tasks 76

SECTION VI: Local Mutual Aid 81
TEMPLATE: Local, Regional, and State Mutual Aid 81
TEMPLATE: Inter-Local Government Agreement–Mutual Aid 83

ANNEX I: Sample Mutual Aid Agreements 89
EXAMPLE: Single County Mutual Aid Agreement 89
EXAMPLE: Single State Mutual Aid Compact 93

ANNEX II: Sample Mass Gathering Event Planning Tools 111
Sample EMS Operations Plan 113
Sample After Action Report 121
Sample Incident Action Plan 127
ANNEX III: Emergency Management Assistance Compact 135
EMAC Operational Considerations 137
ANNEX IV: FEMA National Ambulance Contract 141
FEMA National Ambulance Contract Operational Considerations 143
ANNEX V: Intrastate Mutual Aid System 145
ANNEX VI: National Disaster Medical System-Disaster Medical Assistance Teams 149
ANNEX VII: References 153
References and Reading List 153

Introduction

Project Background

Emergency Medical Services (EMS) agencies regardless of service delivery model have sought guidance on how to better integrate their emergency preparedness and response activities into similar processes occurring at the local, regional, State, tribal and Federal levels. The primary purpose of this project is to begin the process of providing that guidance as it relates to mass care incident deployment.

The World Bank reported in 2005 that on aggregate, the reported number of natural disasters worldwide has been rapidly increasing, from fewer than 100 in 1975 to more than 400 in 2005. Terrorism, pandemic surge, and natural disasters have had a major impact on the science of planning for and responding to mass care incidents and remain a significant threat to the homeland. From the attacks of September 11th, 2001, the subsequent use of anthrax as a biological weapon, to the more recent surge concerns following the outbreak of H1N1 influenza, EMS have a real and immediate need for integration with the emergency management process, and to coordinate efforts with partners across the spectrum of the response community.

The barriers identified from the literature review and interviews with national EMS leadership include:

- lack of access to emergency preparedness grant funding;
- underrepresentation on local, regional, and State level planning committees; and
- lack of systematic mandatory inclusion of all EMS provider types in State, regional, and local emergency plans.

In December 2004, New York University's Center for Catastrophe Preparedness and Response held a national roundtable that included experts from major organizations representing the EMS system as a whole. The report from that meeting concluded that:

> *EMS providers, such as fire departments and hospital-based, commercial, and air ambulance services, ensure that patients receive the medical care they need during a terrorist attack. While EMS personnel, including Emergency Medical Technicians and paramedics, represent roughly one-third of traditional first responders (which also include law enforcement and fire service personnel), the EMS system receives only four percent of first responder funding. If EMS personnel are not prepared for a terrorist attack, their ability to provide medical care and transport to victims of an attack will be compromised. There will be an inadequate medical first response.*

In 2007, the Institute of Medicine in its landmark report *Emergency Medical Services at the Crossroads* issued a recommendation that stated:

> *The Department of Health and Human Services (DHHS), the Department of Homeland Security and the States should elevate emergency and trauma care to a position of parity with other public safety entities in disaster planning and operations.*

Since the time of these reports Federal progress to address these issues has included the creation of the Office of Health Affairs (OHA) within the Department of Homeland Security (DHS), the creation of the Emergency Care Coordination Center (ECCC) within HHS, and the creation of the Federal Interagency Committee on EMS (FICEMS) Preparedness Committee. Outputs from these organizations that have contributed to a more efficient and coordinated integration of EMS into preparedness activity are too numerous to recount here.

In an effort to increase the level of preparedness among EMS agencies, the National Emergency Medical Services Management Association (NEMSMA) approached the DHS and OHA to engage them in a partnership that would provide a greater understanding of the shortfalls in EMS emergency preparedness and provide resources to fill those gaps.

The primary objective of this project is to understand model policies and practices across a spectrum of disciplines and provider types that will lead to a better prepared EMS deployment to mass care incidents. While not a comprehensive guidance document, this project should serve as a foundation for further development of EMS specific policies and templates that improve EMS readiness to manage the full spectrum of hazards that face their communities.

Mass Care Incidents

"Mass Care incident" is defined for the purpose of this publication as any event; planned or unplanned that results in the need to provide medical care to patients outside of traditional hospital settings. Broadly, incidents are divided into planned events (special events—like a sporting event or political protest) and unplanned incidents (such as terrorism, earthquakes, natural disasters, or weather related triggering mechanisms).

Review of Model Policies and Protocols

The Commission on Accreditation of Ambulance Services (CAAS) requires that accredited agencies have some form of policy to address mutual aid and mass casualty deployment. However, in examining several example policies, the focus is on tactical definitions of mass casualty incidents, the number and type of personnel needed to manage those incidents, and boilerplate language regarding compliance with the National Incident Management System (NIMS). Further research is needed to determine the elements of a successful policy that most directly lead to quality management of mass care and mass casualty incidents. A cross section of policies has been included to provide planners with a starting point to develop their own agency level policies regarding mass care and mass incident deployment. These policies come from public and private EMS agencies as well as State offices of EMS.

Document Format

The document provides guidance in the form of usable templates and examples. For the purpose of the document, the term "template" is used both to mean documents that are intended to be filled in with the user's information, as well as a pattern for accomplishing a specific task (operational template). There are several annexes to the document that describe key programs that foster EMS integration into the planning and response process. Those include the Emergency Management Assistance Compact (EMAC), FEMA National Ambulance Contract, and the Interstate Mutual Aid System. Finally the references and resources annex documents provide an excellent reading list as well as a roadmap to the scientific foundations of the document.

Incident Command System

Terminology and concepts of Incident Command are used throughout this document. Further information on Incident Command System (ICS) concepts is available through courses developed by FEMA including:

ICS-100, *Introduction to ICS for Operational First Responders*
ICS-200, *Basic NIMS ICS for Operational First Responders*
ICS-300, *Intermediate ICS for Expanding Incidents for Operational First Responders*
ICS-400, *Advanced ICS for Command and General Staff, Complex Incidents, and MACS*
ICS-402, *Incident Command System (ICS) Overview for Executives/Senior Officials*

References

- Center for Catastrophe Preparedness and Response NYU. "Emergency Medical Services: The Forgotten First Responder–A Report on the Critical Gaps in Organization and Deficits in Resources for America's Medical First Responders." New York: New York University, 2005.

- Institute of Medicine. (2006). *Emergency Medical Services at the Crossroads*. Retrieved from: http://www.iom.edu/Reports/2006/Emergecy-Medical-Services-At-the-Crossroads.aspx

SECTION I: Emergency Medical Services Deployment Templates
TEMPLATE 1: The Emergency Medical Services Emergency Operations Plan

<EMS AGENCY> EOP Overview

The centerpiece of comprehensive emergency management is the emergency operations plan (EOP). The **<EMS AGENCY>** EOP will make use of a variety of sources to ensure compliance with Federal, State, and local planning guidance. The concepts and guidance within the National Incident Management System (NIMS) will be used and referenced to ensure consistency with Incident Command System (ICS) principles and practices. The **<EMS AGENCY>** will develop an EOP that defines the scope of preparedness and incident management activities needed to accomplish its assigned missions. The **<EMS AGENCY>** EOP:

- Assigns responsibility to carry out specific actions at projected times and places during an emergency that exceeds the capability or routine responsibility of any one agency.
- Sets forth lines of authority and organizational relationships and shows how all actions will be coordinated.
- Describes how people and property are protected in emergencies and disasters.
- Identifies personnel, equipment, facilities, supplies, and other resources available—within the jurisdiction or by agreement with other jurisdictions—for use during response and recovery operations.
- Reconciles requirements with other jurisdictions.
- Identifies steps to address mitigation concerns during response and recovery activities.

An EOP is flexible enough for use in all emergencies. A complete EOP describes the:

- purpose of the plan;
- situation;
- assumptions;
- concept of operations (CONOPS);
- organization and assignment of responsibilities;
- administration and logistics;
- plan development and maintenance; and
- authorities and references.

The EOP contains annexes and appendices appropriate to the **<EMS AGENCY>**'s organization and operations. EOPs identify or designate functional area representatives to the Incident Command, Unified Command (UC), or multiagency coordination entity whenever possible to facilitate responsive and collaborative incident management. An EOP also defines the scope of **preparedness** activities necessary to make the EOP more than a mere paper plan. This is because the EOP defines the requirements to effectively manage response. These requirements are used to set training and exercise goals. Training helps emergency personnel become familiar with their responsibilities and acquire the skills necessary to perform assigned tasks. Exercises pro-

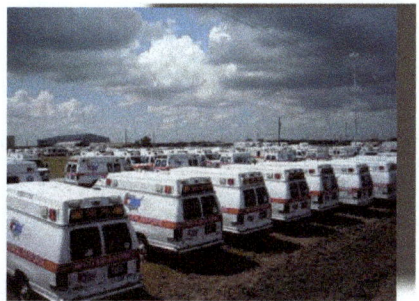

Ambulances responded as part of the critical asset deployment for Hurricane Dean.

vide a means to validate plans, checklists, and response procedures and evaluate the skills of personnel. In addition, exercise can identify gaps in expected performance and outcomes that should be addressed through a variety of mechanisms. Common mechanisms include additional training, updating or adding equipment, incorporating technology, or enhancing existing agreements with response partners.

Adjusting an EOP after conducting training or exercises or responding to events also makes it practice-based. The EOP facilitates **response** and **short-term recovery** (which set the stage for successful **long-term recovery**). Response actions are time-sensitive. Some post disaster recovery issues, such as the rebuilding and placement of temporary housing facilities, also must be addressed quickly. Advance planning makes performing this task easier, especially when a changing environment requires midcourse corrections.

<EMS AGENCY> EOP Outline
Basic Plan

- promulgation document/signature page;
- approval and implementation;
- record of changes;
- table of contents;
- purpose, scope, authority, and analysis;
    - purpose,
    - scope,
    - authority,
    - hazard vulnerability analysis, and
    - capability assessment;
- planning assumptions–employing The Planning P (See diagram on page 19.);
- concept of operations;
- organization and assignment of responsibilities;
- direction, control, and coordination;
- disaster intelligence;
- communications;
- administration, finance, and logistics;
- plan development and maintenance; and
- authorities and references.

Response Partnerships

- fire;
- law enforcement;
- emergency medical services (EMS);
- emergency management;
- Federal agencies;
- hospitals;
- public health agencies;
- public works;
- mass shelter and feeding;
- veterinarians and animal sheltering groups; and
- volunteer and nongovernmental organizations.

Support Agencies

- Identify those agencies that have a support role during an emergency.

TEMPLATE 2: Basic Hazard Vulnerability Analysis

Hazard Vulnerability Analysis for <INSERT JURISDICTION HERE>
<EMS AGENCY>

Introduction

Insert an introduction to the plan here that contains background and methods used to collect information on the hazards present in the local community.

Geographic Characteristics

Geography
Describe any geographic features such as known fault lines, features that result in geographic isolation of one or more parts of the jurisdiction (limited river crossings, mountain passes, etc.).

Climate
Describe the climate by season with a focus on climate conditions that have Emergency Medical Services (EMS) implications such as heat waves, periods of extreme cold, snow, wind hazards, or other weather related data that poses a hazard to the public.

Demographic Characteristics

Economic Factors
Describe the economic situation in the community. Include average income, home prices, occupancy rates, and unemployment at a minimum.

Crime Statistics
Describe the crime rate for crimes against persons and any other special criminal risks (gang activity, narcotics trafficking, etc.) that pose special risk to the jurisdiction.

Specific Hazards

Summary
Summarize the type of hazards present in the jurisdiction. Describe the specific hazards found in the community, natural and/or manmade, using historical data for risk assessment.

Potential Hazards for <INSERT JURISDICTION HERE>
<INSERT HAZARD TYPE HERE>

Describe the type of hazard in detail. Include specific examples of the hazard as it exists in the community. Differentiate between threats and risks in accordance with risk assessment principles.

History

Describe any history of the incident type including the date, time, and recorded consequences of the event.

Potential Impact

Describe potential impacts to the jurisdiction if the incident type should occur. Focus on impacts on EMS service, hospital surge, and need for mass shelter or feeding operations.

Vulnerability

Identify points of vulnerability that result in the potential impacts detailed in the paragraph above.

Probability

Estimate the probability of occurrence for this incident type.

Some common hazard types are listed below along with definitions

Dam Failure: Dam failure may be caused by flooding, earthquakes, poor construction, lack of maintenance and repair, improper operation, or acts of vandalism or terrorism.

Drought: A drought is defined as "a period of abnormally dry weather sufficiently prolonged and severe enough to reduce soil moisture, water and snow levels to drop below the minimum levels necessary to sustain animal, plant and economic systems."

Earthquakes: Earthquakes cause damage by strong ground shaking and by the secondary effects of ground failures and tsunamis. The strength of ground shaking generally decreases with the distance from the earthquake source. Shaking can be much higher when earthquake waves are intensified by bedrock and then pass through softer earth materials such as sediment. Ground failures caused by earthquakes include fault rupture, ground cracking, landslides, rock fall, liquefaction and uplift. Faults do not often rupture through to the surface. Unstable ground is mostly at risk of the other effects. Any of these failures will affect structures above or below them.

Epidemic: Epidemics are outbreaks of disease that affect, or threaten to affect, a significant portion of a population in a relatively short period of time. Although usually referring to human contagious disease, epidemics can also affect domestic and wild animals and crops. Epidemic diseases are usually introduced into an area from remote regions and inflict devastation because there is no natural or induced immunity.

Forest Fires/Wildfires: A forest fire is considered as any uncontrolled burning within a forested area and uncontrolled and hard to extinguish burning in grassland, brush or woodland.

Flooding: Groundwater flooding occurs when the water table is high and there is persistent heavy rain. Water collects in any natural depression when the soil can no longer absorb the water.

Hazardous Material: Chemical hazards are created when there is a release of toxic agents into the atmosphere and environment that can harm population, animals, and food supplies.

Heat Waves: A heat wave is characterized by five or more consecutive days of unusually hot weather.

Landslide/Erosion: The term landslide refers to the downward movement of a slope and masses of rock, soil or other debris under the force of gravity. Slides range in size from thin masses of soil a few yards wide to deep-seated bedrock slides. The form of initial failure commonly categorizes slides, but they may travel in a variety of forms along their paths. This travel rate may range in velocity from a few inches per month to many feet per second, depending largely on slope, material and water content.

Erosion refers to the gradual removal of soil through wind or water action. Erosion may be induced or increased by failure to use ground covers to protect soil from wind or drainage systems to allow good dispersal of storm water. Slopes on waterfront can also be severely undercut by normal water flow, wave action or large waves produced by storms.

Nuclear Incidents: Nuclear incidents result from a release of radioactive material into the atmosphere from sources such as nuclear power facilities, military installations that house nuclear powered vessels, or nuclear storage facilities.

Storm: Destructive storms come in several forms: wind, rain, ice, snow, and a combination. Any winter storm can pack high winds and heavy rain causing widespread damage. High winds of short duration, such as tornadoes and strong gusts from thunderstorms, can also be destructive though generally not as widespread.

Terrorism: Terrorism is defined as the use of force or violence against persons or property violating the criminal laws of the United States for purposes of intimidation, coercion, or ransom. Terrorists often use threats to create fear among the public for the purpose of influencing political process and generate publicity. Terrorism can be broken down further into chemical, biological, radiological, nuclear, explosive, and cyber related forms of attack. Mass shooting incidents can also be a form of terrorism based upon motivation and intent.

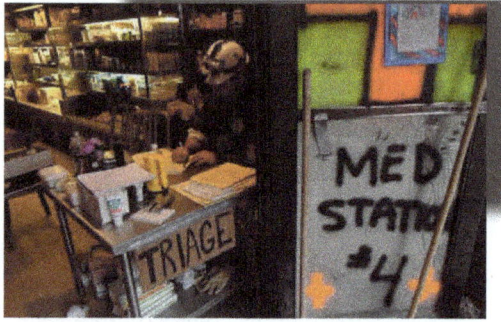

Triage station near the sight of the World Trade Center after the terrorist attacks of September 11, 2011.

Tsunami/High Waves/Seiches: Tsunamis are sea waves generated by seismic activity, underwater volcanic eruptions, meteor impacts, or landslides.

Volcanoes/Ash Fall: Volcanic eruptions can cause damage through direct exposure to eruption materials (lava, etc.) or by ash fall. The probability of ash fall depends on wind direction and the volcanic source of the eruption causing the ash fall. Most of the dangers are to persons in the near vicinity of the volcano. Other dangers, such as mudflows and ash fall, may exist miles downstream and down wind.

References

- Endsley, M.R. 1995. "Toward a Theory of Situation Awareness in Dynamic Systems." *The Journal of the Human Factors and Ergonomics Society* 31 (1): 32-64.

- Woodbury, G.L. "Washington State Hazard Identification and Vulnerability Assessment." Washington Emergency Management Division, (2005): 16-24.

TEMPLATE 3: Incident and Event Plans

All events and incidents **<EMS AGENCY>** participates in will have an Event Plan for planned events, an Incident Action Plan (IAP) for unplanned events, or both.

Event and Incident Planning Process

Refer to the chart below for information on the Command and General staff members' responsibilities for planning.

Incident Commander	• Provides overall incident objectives and strategy.
	 • Establishes procedures for incident resource ordering.
	 • Establishes procedures for resource activation, mobilization, and employment.
	 • Approves completed IAP by signature.
	 • With Safety Officer:
	    − Reviews hazards associated with the incident and proposed tactical assignments.
	    − Assists in developing safe tactics.
	    − Develops safety message(s).

Operations Section Chief	• Assists in identifying strategies. • Determines tactics to achieve command objectives. • Determines work assignments and resource requirements.
Planning Section Chief	• Conducts the Planning Meeting. • Coordinates preparation and documentation of the IAP.
Logistics Section Chief	• Ensures that resource ordering procedures are communicated to appropriate agency ordering points. • Develops a transportation system to support operational needs. • Ensures that the Logistics Section can support the IAP. • Completes assigned portions of the written IAP. • Places order(s) for resources. • Ensures that responders receive operational medical care when needed.
Finance/Admin. Section Chief	• Provides cost implications of incident objectives, as required. • Ensures that the IAP is within the financial limits established by the Incident Commander (IC). • Evaluates facilities, transportation assets, and other contracted services to determine if any special contract arrangements are needed.

- Incident objectives should be developed that cover the entire course of the incident. For complex incidents, it may take more than one operational period to accomplish the incident objectives.

- The cyclical planning process is designed to take the overall incident objectives and break them down into tactical assignments for each operational period. It is important that this initial overall approach to establishing incident objectives establish the course of the incident, rather than having incident objectives only address a single operational period.

- The incident objectives must conform to the legal obligations and management objectives of all affected agencies.

Sound, timely planning provides the foundation for effective incident management. The National Incident Management System (NIMS) planning process represents a template for strategic, operational, and tactical planning that includes all steps an IC and other members of the Command and General Staffs should take to develop and disseminate an IAP. The planning process may begin with the scheduling of a planned event, the identification of a credible threat, or with the initial response to an actual or impending event. The process continues with the implementation of the formalized steps and staffing required in developing a written IAP. A clear, concise IAP is essential to guide the initial incident management decision process and the continuing collective planning activities of incident management teams. The planning process should provide the following:

- current information that accurately describes and assesses the incident situation and resource status;

- predictions of the probable course of events;

- alternative strategies to attain critical incident objectives; and

- an accurate, realistic IAP for the next operational period.

The following five primary phases must be followed, in sequence, to ensure a comprehensive IAP:

1. Understand the situation.

2. Establish incident objectives and strategy.

3. Develop the IAP.

4. Prepare and disseminate the IAP.

5. Evaluate and revise the plan.

Operational Planning Cycle

The IAP must provide clear strategic direction and include a comprehensive listing of the tactical objectives, resources, reserves, and support required to accomplish each overarching incident objective. The comprehensive IAP will state the sequence of events in a coordinated way for achieving multiple incident objectives. However, the IAP is based on the best available information at the time of the planning meeting. Planning meetings should not be delayed in anticipation of future information.

During the initial stages of incident management, planners must develop a simple plan that can be communicated through concise oral briefings. Frequently, this plan must be developed very quickly and with incomplete situation information. As the incident management effort evolves over time, additional lead time, staff, information systems, and technologies will enable more detailed planning and cataloging of events and "lessons learned."

The Planning "P"

- Preparing for the Planning Meeting
- Planning Meeting
- IAP Prep and Approval
- Tactics Meeting
- Operations Briefing
- New Start Ops Period Begins
- IC/UC Sets Objectives
- Execute Plan and Assess Progress
- Initial IC/UC Meeting
- Operational Period Planning Cycle
- Incident Briefing ICS 201
- Initial Response and Assessment
- Notification
- Incident/Threat

The leg of the "P" describes the initial response period: Once the incident/threat begins, the steps are Notification, Initial Response and Assessment, Incident Briefing (ICS Form 201), and Initial Incident Command and, if necessary, expansion to a Unified Command (UC) Meeting.

At the top of the leg of the "P" is the beginning of the first operational planning period cycle. In this circular sequence, the steps are: Incident Command/UC Sets the Incident Objectives, Tactics Meeting, Preparing for the Planning Meeting, Planning Meeting, IAP Prep and Approval, and Operations Briefing.

At this point, a new operations period begins. The next step is Execute Plan and Assess Progress, after which the cycle begins anew with Incident Command/UC Sets Objectives.

Before each operational period begins, the incident objectives must be assessed and updated as needed. Ask the following questions:

- Is the incident stable, or is it increasing in size and complexity?
- What are the current incident objectives, strategy, and tactics?
- Are there any safety issues?
- Are the objectives effective? Is a change of course needed?
- How long will it be until the objectives are completed?
- What is the current status of resources? Are resources in good condition? Are there sufficient resources?

Tactics Meetings

The purpose of the tactics meeting is to review the tactics developed by the Operations Section Chief. This includes:

- Determining how the selected strategy will be accomplished in order to achieve the incident objectives.
- Assigning resources to implement the tactics.
- Identifying methods for monitoring tactics and resources to determine if adjustments are required (e.g., different tactics, different resources, or new strategy).
- The Operations Section Chief, Safety Officer, Planning Section Chief, Logistics Section Chief, and Resources Unit Leader attend the tactics meeting.
- The Operations Section Chief leads the tactics meeting. The ICS Form 215, Operational Planning Worksheet, is used to document the tactics meeting.

Determining Tactics

Incident objectives state what is to be accomplished in the operational period. Make use of the SMART objective development process:

S–Specific: Is the incident objective wording precise and unambiguous?

M–Measurable: How will achievements be measured?

A–Action Oriented: Is an action verb used to describe the expected accomplishments?

R–Realistic: Is the outcome achievable with give available resources?

T–Time Sensitive: What is the timeframe in which the activity is to occur?

Strategies establish the general plan or direction for accomplishing the incident objectives.
Tactics specify how the strategies will be executed.

Developing Strategy

The Operational Section Chief generates alternative strategies to meet the incident objectives that:

- Are within acceptable safety norms.
- Make sense (is feasible, practical, and suitable).
- Are cost effective.
- Are consistent with sound environmental practices.
- Meet political considerations.

Tactical Direction

- Tactical direction describes what must be accomplished within the selected strategy or strategies in order to achieve the incident objectives. Tactical direction is the responsibility of the IC or the Operations Section Chief (if that position has been assigned by the IC).
- The IC or the Operations Section Chief gathers input from the Branch Directors and Division and/or Group Supervisors on alternative tactics. Jointly developed tactics can ensure understanding and enhance commitment.
- Tactical direction consists of the following steps:
  - **Establish Tactics:** Determine the tactics needed to implement the selected strategy. Typically, tactics are to be accomplished within an operational period. During more complex incidents, tactical direction should be stated in terms of accomplishments that can realistically be achieved within the timeframe currently being planned.
  - **Assign Resources:** Determine and assign the kind and type of resources appropriate for the selected tactics. Resource assignments will consist of the kind, type, and numbers of resources available and needed to achieve the tactical operations desired for the operational period.
  - **Monitor Performance:** Performance monitoring will determine if the tactics and resources selected for the various strategies are both valid and adequate.

TEMPLATE 4: Basic Incident Deployment Checklists

<EMS AGENCY> Basic Deployment Checklists
Accountability Procedures

- **Check-In.**

    All responders, regardless of agency affiliation, must check-in to verify their assignment. This can be coordinated by using an Incident Check-In List (ICS Form 211).

- **Incident Action Plan (IAP) Compliance.**

    <EMS AGENCY> incident/event operations must be directed and coordinated as outlined in the IAP. Any deviation must be approved by the Operations Chief and communicated to and approved by the Incident Commander (IC). **<EMS AGENCY>** personnel accountability procedures should be documented within the IAP.

- **Unity of Command.**

    In order to prevent accountability breakdowns, each individual operating on behalf of **<EMS AGENCY>** involved in incident management will be assigned to only one supervisor.

- **Span of Control.**

    Supervisors must be able to adequately supervise, communicate with, manage and control all personnel under their supervision. Span of control may vary between 3 and 7 personnel per supervisor, with a recommended ratio of 1 to 5.

- **Resource Tracking.**

    Supervisors must record resource status changes as they occur and report those changes to the Resources Unit. Accountability is dependent upon the incident management organization having a standard resource tracking method.

Common Responsibilities

The following checklist is applicable to all **<EMS AGENCY>** personnel operating in an Incident Command System (ICS):

❏ Upon arrival at the incident, check-in at one of the following designated check-in locations:
- Incident Command Post (ICP);
- Base;
- Staging Areas; and
- Other area designated by the Incident Command.

Note: If instructed to report directly to a tactical assignment, check-in with the Division/Group Supervisor or the Operations Section Chief in charge of the area of operations.

❏ Receive briefing from immediate supervisor and document briefing on a Unit Log (ICS Form 214).

UNIT LOG	1. Incident Name	2. Date Prepared	3. Time Prepared
4. Unit Name/Designators	5. Unit Leader (Name and Position)		6. Operational Period

7. Roster of Assigned Personnel		
Name	ICS Position	Home Base

8. Activity Log	
Time	Major Events

9. Prepared by (Name and Position)

- Acquire work materials.
- Abide by organizational code of ethics, policies, procedures, and applicable labor agreements.
- Participate in Incident Management Team (IMT) meetings and briefings as appropriate.
- Ensure compliance with all safety practices and procedures. Report unsafe conditions to the Safety Officer (SO).
- Supervisors: Maintain accountability for assigned personnel with regard to exact location(s), personal safety, and welfare at all times, especially when working in or around incident operations.
- Supervisors: Organize and brief subordinates.
- Know the assigned communication methods and procedures for the Area of Responsibility (AOR) and ensure that communications equipment is operating properly.
- Use plain language and ICS terminology (no codes) in all radio communications.
- Complete forms, reports, and ICS Form 214 that are required of the assigned position and ensure proper disposition of incident documentation as directed by the Documentation Unit.
- Ensure all equipment is operational prior to each work period.
- Report any signs/symptoms of extended incident stress, injury, fatigue, or illness to a supervisor.
- Brief shift replacement about ongoing operations when relieved at operational periods or during rotation.
- Respond to demobilization orders and brief subordinates regarding demobilization.
- Prepare personal belongings for demobilization.
- Complete demobilization check-out process before being released from the incident, including the return of all equipment.
- Upon demobilization, report estimated time of arrival (ETA) to home agency.
- Participate in after-action activities as directed.

Leadership Responsibilities

In National Incident Management System (NIMS) ICS, a number of the leadership responsibilities are common to all functions within the ICS organization. Common responsibilities of Unit Leaders are listed below.

Medical Branch Director: The Medical Branch Director is responsible for the implementation of the IAP within the Branch. This includes the direction and execution of branch planning for the assignment of resources within the Branch. The Branch Director reports to the Operations Section Chief and supervises the Triage, Treatment, and Patient Transportation Group Supervisors as well as the Medical Supply Coordinator. The Medical Branch establishes command and controls the activities within the Medical Area in order to assure the best possible emergency medical care to patients during a multicasualty incident.

- Review Common Responsibilities.
- Review Group/Division Assignments for effectiveness of current operations and modify as needed.
- Provide input to Operations Section Chief for the IAP.
- Supervise Branch activities.
- Report to Operations Section Chief on Branch activities.
- Coordinate with the agency's Medical Director, if available.
- Maintain ICS Form 214.
- Participate in the development of the IAP and review the general control objectives including alternate strategies as appropriate.
- Designate Group Supervisors and Treatment Area locations as appropriate.

Section I: Emergency Medical Services Deployment Templates

- ❏ Recommend Treatment Area locations as appropriate. Isolate Morgue (black) and Minor (green) Treatment Areas away from Immediate (Red) and Delayed (Yellow) Treatment Areas.
- ❏ Consider use of a contaminated patient treatment area (Blue). Determine how to differentiate between contaminated and decontaminated patients.
- ❏ Request law enforcement/Medical Examiner involvement as needed.
- ❏ Collect, review, and compile casualty information.
- ❏ Recommend additional personnel and resources sufficient to handle the magnitude of the incident.
- ❏ Determine amount and types of additional medical resources and supplies needed to handle the magnitude of the incident (medical caches, backboards, litters, cots).
- ❏ Establish communications and coordination with Patient Transportation Group Supervisor.
- ❏ Ensure activation of hospital alert system, local EMS/health agencies.
- ❏ Direct and/or supervise on scene personnel from agencies such as Medical Examiner's Office, Red Cross, law enforcement, private ambulance companies, county health agencies, and hospital volunteers.
- ❏ Ensure proper security, traffic control, and access for the area.
- ❏ Direct medically trained personnel in coordination with the appropriate Treatment Group Supervisor.
- ❏ Maintain ICS Form 214.

Triage Group Supervisor: The Triage Group Supervisor reports to the Medical Branch Director and supervises Triage Personnel/Litter Bearers and the Morgue Unit Leader. The Triage Group Supervisor assumes responsibility for providing triage management and movement of patients from the triage area. When triage has been completed, the Group Supervisor may be reassigned as needed.

- ❏ Review Common Responsibilities.
- ❏ Review Group Supervisor Responsibilities.
- ❏ Develop organization sufficient to handle assignment.
- ❏ Inform Medical Branch Director of resource needs.
- ❏ Implement triage process.
- ❏ Coordinate movement of patients from the Triage Area (incident site) to the appropriate Treatment Area.
- ❏ Give periodic status reports to Medical Branch Director.
- ❏ Maintain security and control of the Triage Area.
- ❏ Establish Morgue with Medical Examiner personnel when possible.
- ❏ Establish area for contaminated casualties if necessary.

Treatment Group Supervisor: The Treatment Group Supervisor reports to the Medical Branch Director and supervises the Treatment Unit Leaders and the Treatment Dispatch Unit Leader. The Treatment Group Supervisor assumes responsibility for treatment, preparation for transport, and coordination of patient treatment in the Treatment Areas and directs movement of patients to loading location(s).

- ❏ Review Common Responsibilities.
- ❏ Review Unit Leader Responsibilities.
- ❏ Develop organization sufficient to handle assignment.
- ❏ Direct and supervise Treatment Dispatch, Immediate (Red), Delayed (Yellow), Minor (Green), Contaminated (Blue) Treatment Areas.
- ❏ Coordinate movement of patients from Triage Area to Treatment Areas with Triage Unit Leader.
- ❏ Request sufficient medical caches and supplies as necessary.

- ❏ Establish communications and coordination with Patient Transportation Group.
- ❏ Ensure continual triage of patients throughout Treatment Areas.
- ❏ Direct movement of patients to ambulance loading area(s).
- ❏ Give periodic status reports to Medical Branch Director.

Patient Transportation Group Supervisor: Transportation Group Supervisor reports to the Medical Branch Director and supervises the Medical Communications Coordinator and Air and Ground Ambulance Coordinators. This supervisor is responsible for the coordination of patient transportation and maintenance of records relating to patient identification, injuries, mode of off-incident transportation, and destination.

- ❏ Review Common Responsibilities.
- ❏ Establish communications with hospital(s).
- ❏ Designate ambulance staging areas(s).
- ❏ Direct the transportation of patients as determined by Treatment Group Supervisor or Unit Leaders.
- ❏ Assure that patient information and destination is recorded.
- ❏ Establish communications with Ambulance Coordinator(s).
- ❏ Request additional ambulances, as required.
- ❏ Notify Ambulance Coordinator(s) of ambulance requests.
- ❏ Coordinate requests for air ambulance transportation through the Air Operations Director.
- ❏ Establish air ambulance landing zone with the Medical Branch Director and Air Operations Director.
- ❏ Maintain ICS Form 214.

References

- Federal Emergency Management Agency. "ICS-300: Intermediate ICS for Expanding Incidents (EMI Course Number: G300)." Emergency Management Institute, 2011.

- Federal Emergency Management Agency. "ICS All Hazards Core Competencies." Emergency Management Institute, 2011.

SECTION II: Mass Care Coordination Toolkit

Introduction to the Coordination Planning Toolkit

This collection of operational templates is intended to assist Emergency Medical Services (EMS) personnel in planning for, responding to, and recovering from a representative assortment of scenarios that could impact their operations. An emphasis is placed on coordinating effectively with other agencies that may also be involved in the response. This toolkit is intended as a starting point, is not comprehensive, and must be adjusted for geographical, logistical, and political considerations.

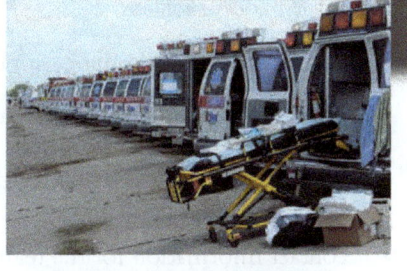

Ambulances are staged and ready to help residents as a hurricane approaches.

Preestablished mutual aid agreements are considered essential for effective response to and recovery from EMS incidents. The following scenarios will be used to illustrate various planning, response, and recovery situations:

- local high school football game;
- residential medical facility evacuation;
- county fair;
- large, participatory sporting event (marathon, ironman, etc.);
- weather-related disaster declaration;
- large college sporting event;
- political assembly;
- auto racing/competition; and
- cancer walk.

High School Football Game

Prepare

Preparing for a local, low-visibility sporting event such as a high school football game begins with collecting information such as:

- requesting agency, point of contact, and contact information for follow-up;
- financial compensation information, if applicable;
- location of event(s) including intended staging location of ambulance and crew, ingress and egress routes from field;
- contact information for the teams athletic trainer/sports medicine personnel if applicable;
- contact information for any security or event personnel involved; and
- anticipated/historical attendance numbers, issues.

When this information has been obtained, a very brief risk assessment should be performed (if one has not already been done for this type of event). Contact should be made with any other involved medical personnel to coordinate operations:

- Athletic trainers
    - Athletic trainers may be able to assist with injured players.
    - Athletic trainers may be trained in cardiopulmonary resuscitation (CPR)/automated external defibrillator (AED) and are likely to be first on scene if a player collapses.
    - Can assist with removing protective equipment, such as helmets.
- Sports medicine staff
    - Sports medicine staff will be able to assist with injured players.
    - Sports medicine staff should be trained in CPR/AED and are likely to arrive before EMS.
- Security staff
    - Security staff may have CPR/AED training and should know where AEDs are located at the event. Security staff will be helpful in locating or moving ill or injured spectators.
    - Security staff will also be able to help in guiding additional medical resources to the incident.
- Fire department or EMS agency (if different from your own) that has jurisdiction over the location of the event.
    - If your agency does not have jurisdiction, the agency with jurisdiction may choose to respond and assume control of any incident that occurs.

Additional Resources:

- National Athletic Trainers' Association.
- Your State's Athletic Trainers' Association.

- American Medical Society for Sports Medicine.
- American College of Sports Medicine.
- National Academy of Sports Medicine.
- American Orthopedic Society for Sports Medicine.
- American Medical Athletic Association.
- County medical association.
- Local volunteer groups.

Forms:
- When coordinating planning with other agencies, an ICS Form 201 (Incident Briefing) should be sufficient.
- If ICS forms are going to address other disciplines such as security or logistics, add an ICS Form 206 (Medical Plan).

Respond

Responding to an emergency at any spectator sport will become a high-visibility event. Inevitably, photos and video of the responding personnel will be available on the internet within minutes of the incident occurring. A Public Information Officer (PIO) should be appointed.

If an event occurs in the stands, parking lot, or other areas, security and other event personnel might not be aware of the emergency. This is where the EMS planning related to collection of contact information will become useful. Communication personnel can use the contact information to notify event staff as well as direct them to acquire an AED or other equipment if applicable.

For incidents involving multiple agencies, a copy of the completed ICS Form 201 can help to orient the Incident Commander (IC) to the area and resources available. Additional ICS forms may be used in the Incident Action Plan (IAP) based on the type and scope of incident.

Recover

Recovery from this type of event should not be overly complex. Recovery will likely be limited to cleaning and restocking equipment according to standard operating procedures (SOPs). In instances involving emotionally charged situations, such as unsuccessful resuscitation of a child, debriefing or Critical Incident Stress Management (CISM) may be indicated. If issues arose during the response or patient treatment that have attracted the attention of conventional or social media, a PIO needs to be appointed for the incident and active management of the situation should begin.

If the incident involves numerous units or lasts several hours, demobilization procedures should be followed and recorded on ICS Form 221 (Demobilization) to ensure that mutual aid and other resources are properly accounted for and returned to service.

Residential Medical Facility Evacuation

Prepare

Preparations for evacuation of a residential medical facility such as a nursing home or senior-citizen center should be taken very seriously. Any large evacuation of a vulnerable population such as this is likely to result in some injuries or exacerbated illness. Responders are at increased risk of injuries due to repetitive lifting in a high-stress situation. Residents are at risk of being injured during moves. The extra activity and stress of an evacuation may result in respiratory, cardiovascular, or other medical complications.

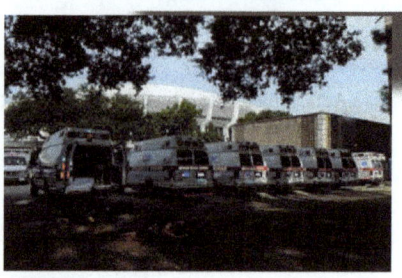

Ambulances await calls during an evacuation of patients with special needs.

A risk assessment should be performed for your community to determine which facilities are at highest risk for evacuation. This would include facilities vulnerable to wildfire, earthquake, flooding and other weather-related threats. A majority of planning resources should be devoted to these facilities, although evacuation due to fire or utility failure can occur anywhere.

Evacuation planning should be conducted in coordination with numerous agencies and individuals:

- Decisionmakers from the involved facility.
  - Background information such as average census, location of the most vulnerable residents, etc.
  - Information on what type of evacuation equipment might be available, such as stair chairs and evacuation mattresses and where it is stored or obtained in an emergency.
  - Responsible for securing receiving facilities for residents during a precautionary evacuation.
  - Responsible for providing training to their staff on the evacuation procedures.
  - Copies of the facility floor plan outlining exits and locations of emergency equipment.
- Fire department and police department.
  - Fire department may provide additional personnel even if no immediate life-threats exist.
  - Police department may assist with controlling traffic or provide additional personnel.
- Emergency management.
  - Will likely provide the information that triggers decisionmakers at the involved facility to begin a precautionary evacuation.
  - In some situations, officials may order a mandatory evacuation.
  - Able to coordinate resources to assist with the evacuation.
- Public health department.
  - May be able to assist in coordination process.
  - May have access to medical assets such as Medical Reserve Corps or Metropolitan Medical Response System.

- Decisionmakers from facilities that might be asked to receive residents from the evacuated facility.
  - May have special restrictions or instructions for receiving residents.
- Mutual aid partners.
  - Verify that your mutual aid partners will honor a request for aid if it involves a precautionary evacuation, with no immediate emergency.
- Area EMS agencies.
  - Determine type and number of resources that are likely to be available from each agency.
  - Estimate time to respond based on location of base of operations.
- Transportation services.
  - Wheelchair van services.
  - School buses.
  - Public buses.
  - Taxi services.
- American Red Cross.
  - May be involved in coordinating sheltering in the case of an emergency evacuation or if insufficient receiving facilities can be identified for the evacuees.
- Salvation Army.
  - May be involved in providing food or other assistance to temporary shelters.
- National Guard, Medical Reserve Corps, National Disaster Medical System, Metropolitan Medical Response System.
  - These assets are unlikely to be helpful due to time needed to respond but may be useful if advance warning of an evacuation available.

Additional Resources:
- National Fire Protection Association—"Emergency Evacuation Planning Guide for People with Disabilities."
- National Disaster Medical System personnel have extensive experience setting up temporary medical facilities.
- Department of Health and Human Services website is an excellent source of information pertaining to facility evacuations.

An ICS Form 201 could be used to document planning for a facility evacuation, or a custom operations template might be used. An ICS Form 215a (Incident Action Plan Safety and Risk Analysis) could be used to document specific hazards within the building such as hazardous chemicals or bulk oxygen storage.

Respond

When requested to respond to a residential medical facility evacuation, it is important to clearly define roles and responsibilities. Typically, facility staff are responsible for all activities within the facility such as obtaining admission for the residents at another facility and determining which patients should be transported first.

Similarly, the EMS service with jurisdiction in the area typically is responsible for residents once they exit the facility. This includes organizing the loading of buses, ambulances, and other forms of transportation. However, in a precautionary evacuation situation, facility staff may take on responsibility for organizing all transports if they have sufficient staff and resources. Regardless of how the incident is organized, EMS personnel must work very closely with facility staff to ensure that each resident is transported safely to the appropriate destination.

Additional complexities will be involved in an emergency evacuation. An emergency evacuation will likely be very personnel intensive and physically demanding, especially in a facility with no or limited elevator availability. Evacuations involving stairways are especially demanding and will require more personnel than evacuations at a single-level facility.

A facility evacuation will likely attract the attention of media and will involve concerned family members. Therefore, appointing a PIO is important.

An incident such as this will likely require ICS Forms 202 (Incident Objective), 203 (Organization Assignment List), 204 (Assignment List), 205 (Incident Radio Communications Plan), and 206 (Medical Plan) as part of the IAP.

Recover
Recovery from a facility evacuation may take many days. It is important for reimbursement purposes that EMS personnel keep excellent records of every transport they provide and any costs associated with the incident. Transportation must be arranged for each resident back to the facility if the building is determined to be safe to occupy. If the facility suffered sufficient damage, the residents may need to be relocated to more permanent facilities while awaiting repair of their home.

For protracted or complex events, ICS Form 221 may be warranted.

County Fair

Prepare

Planning for a county fair or similar outdoor event should begin well in advance and will require planners to decide if the event will require fixed aid stations. Fixed aid stations may be used to provide simple first aid supplies such as band aids, over the counter medications, and hydration drinks. It is important that aid station personnel have protocols approved by their medical director that provide guidance on how to handle nontransport situations that often occur with aid stations.

A simple risk assessment should be performed (if not already performed for this type of event) to determine the likely emergencies responders will encounter.

Preparing for a local, medium-visibility event such as a county fair will require collecting information such as:

- requesting agency, point of contact, contact information for follow-up information;
- financial compensation information if applicable;
- location of event(s) including intended staging location of ambulance and crew, ingress and egress routes;
- contact information for any security or event personnel involved; and
- anticipated/historical attendance numbers, issues.

When this information has been obtained, a very brief risk assessment should be performed (if one has not already been done for this type of event).

- Decisionmakers from the event organizer.
    - Background information such as average attendance, high-risk areas, etc.
    - Responsible for providing training to their staff on the emergency procedures.
    - A map or diagram showing how the event will be laid out, including exits and any obstacles to access or egress.
    - Coordinate location of aid stations.
- Fire department and police department.
    - Fire department may be needed for extrication or rescue situations.
    - Fire inspectors will be involved in ensuring safe conditions for the event participants.
- Event security personnel.
    - Provide assistance locating 9-1-1 callers at the event.
    - May have access to AEDs.
    - Provide assistance directing other emergency crews into the event during an emergency.
- EMS service with jurisdiction if different.

- Veterinarians.
    - Ensure that EMS personnel know how to contact the veterinarian in an emergency.
    - Injured animals may threaten the safety of EMS personnel as well as spectators.
- Mutual aid partners.
    - Make sure mutual aid partners are aware of the event.
    - Coordinate ingress and egress routes should a mutual aid response become necessary.
- Department of Public Health.
    - May be able to assist in providing staff for aid stations.
    - Will be involved in ensuring food safety and sanitation at the event.

The following information sources may be helpful during planning for these events:

- American Veterinary Medical Association.
- Department of Public Health–Food Safety.

At a minimum, ICS Forms 201 and 206 should be included in the IAP.

Respond

Events such as these can produce a broad range of injuries, from dehydration to animal bites. Use extreme caution when operating near livestock or other animals. Sirens may provoke panic in some animals and endanger personnel and participants. Fairs are often spread out over a large area and may necessitate coordination with event personnel to ensure ambulances are parked as close as possible to the patient. In addition, rough or muddy ground may necessitate alternative patient movement techniques.

Mass casualty situations occurring at events such as these can usually be handled with conventional procedures, using additional caution around livestock. As with all mass casualty events, media attention and concerned family members will likely be present. Therefore, a PIO should be appointed.

Recover

Recovery from a mass casualty situation at an event such as this may necessitate extensive cleaning of equipment soiled with dirt or mud. Other unique recovery steps are unlikely.

Marathon or Similar Running Events

Road races such as marathons, half marathons, and shorter events often occur over a very large road course. Although fixed aid stations may be required, means of responding to incidents on the course are also necessary. Caution must be exercised during response to avoid injury to participants or spectators while attempting to respond alongside the runners or attempting to cross a closed course.

Please note that runners in a crowd may not notice an ambulance attempting to cross the course due to the other runners in front of them blocking their vision and the loud background noises from cheering spectators blocking their ability to hear warning devices.

A simple risk assessment should be performed (if not already performed for this type of event) to determine the likely emergencies responders will encounter.

Prepare
- Event sponsor:
  - Determine exact route of course, including road closures and potential emergency crossing points.
  - Determine expected attendance for both participants and spectators. (Participants are much more likely than spectators to request assistance during the event).
  - Determine number and capabilities of medical aid stations for the event. EMS personnel may or may not be involved in staffing/operating the aid stations.
  - Determine the number and type of EMS resources needed.
  - Determine number and qualifications of aid station personnel needed.
- Law enforcement:
  - Coordinate ambulance ingress and egress routes to ensure timely responses and participant and spectator safety.
  - Frequent requestors of medical aid on behalf of spectators or participants. Officers should be provided instructions on what information dispatch requires in order to determine the patient's priority.
- Aid station staff (if different agency providing):
  - Coordinate ambulance ingress and egress.
  - Discuss parameters by which patients will be treated at the aid station, and who will be transported to a hospital.
  - Discuss how to handle moving participants from the course to the aid station.
  - Determine whether EMS will be responsible for providing any supplies to the aid station.
- Representative from local hospitals:
  - Provide information to local hospitals so they can make informed staffing decisions for the day of the race.

- Mutual aid partners, local EMS agencies:
  - Attempt to determine how many additional resources mutual aid partners and local EMS agencies may be able to send in case of a mass care incident.
  - Make sure mutual aid partners are aware of the race and how it will affect traffic/road closures.
  - Events such as these often cross multiple jurisdictions, event planning should incorporate representatives from each jurisdiction, and Unified Command (UC) will likely be necessary.

Additional Resources:
- American Medical Athletic Association.
- American Road Race Medical Society.
- National Athletic Trainers' Association.
- Your State's Athletic Trainers' Association.
- American Medical Society for Sports Medicine.
- American College of Sports Medicine.
- National Academy of Sports Medicine.
- American Orthopedic Society for Sports Medicine.
- American Medical Athletic Association.
- County/Local medical society.
- Local volunteer groups.

ICS Forms 201, 202, 203, 205, 206, and 214 (Unit Log) may all be necessary during planning or response for this type of event. An alternative patient contact form may be considered for some units/situations.

Respond

Units responding to this type of event may be requested to stage a short distance away from the patient while event personnel package and move the patient to the waiting ambulance by stretcher or specialty golf-cart style vehicles. It is critical that all ambulances responding to an event such as this are provided with SOPs guiding whether or not they are permitted to transport patients to the medical aid station.

Recover

Recovery from any mass casualty incident (MCI) is likely to generate a media response, but media will likely already be on site due to their coverage of the event. Assigning a PIO early will help to manage this. If any of the medical aid stations become involved in providing care during a mass casualty situation, it is likely that some mixing of equipment and supplies may occur that needs to be addressed to return units to service.

Weather-Related Disaster Declaration

Disaster declarations caused by weather events such as hurricanes, flooding, tornados, or snow and ice storms require a few unique planning considerations. Weather events frequently affect your mutual aid partners in the same way that your jurisdiction is being affected. Therefore, mutual aid assets that might be available during a mass casualty situation may no longer be available or may not be able to respond to specific areas due to road conditions. This requires EMS services to ensure they have sufficient surge capacity to deal with likely occurrences in their area of operation.

Prepositioning of supplies, personnel, and other resources may be necessary to avoid response interruptions to areas that may be cut off by rising floodwaters, deep snow, or other weather-related barriers. Careful coordination between adjacent municipalities will help to ensure resources are used efficiently.

An indepth risk assessment is critical to planning for these types of events. This risk assessment will require coordination with area Emergency Management officials.

Prepare

Planning for such an extensive event may require coordination with:

- Emergency Management officials.
  - Conduit to political leaders.
  - Coordinate professional risk assessments.
  - Establish an Emergency Operations Center (EOC) during the event.
- Fire department and law enforcement agencies with jurisdiction.
  - EMS ambulances may be stationed at fire stations or police stations to aid in coordination and provide for crew safety.
- Volunteer organizations such as American Red Cross, Salvation Army, etc.
  - Feeding and sheltering of displaced residents likely to be accomplished by one of these two groups.
  - EMS crews are often approached about how to find these shelters so they must have current contact information and location of each shelter.
- Any groups or facilities establishing shelters.
- National Guard.
  - May be a resource for disasters declared in advance of an approaching storm.
  - May be able to provide assistance responding to requests in areas not accessible by ambulance.
- Animal shelter volunteers.
  - Shelter for pets is important for the peace of mind of displaced residents.
- Public Health Department.
  - May be able to provide information on vulnerable populations.
  - May be able to provide access to additional medical personnel via Medical Reserve Corps or other avenues.

- Emergency Management Assistance Compact (EMAC). (See Annex III for additional information.)
  - If facility evacuations or other medical transportation issues exceed the capabilities of State resources, State officials will use EMAC agreements to request additional resources from other States.
- Off-road vehicle clubs.
  - With careful management, volunteers with off-road capable vehicles may be useful for assisting in transporting emergency personnel to scenes inaccessible to conventional response vehicles.
  - Volunteers may be able to assist emergency responders that become stuck in snow or mud.
  - Volunteers may be able to move equipment or personnel from site to site.
- Public Works Department.
  - Public works personnel and equipment will be critical during and after weather-related events.
  - Snow or debris removal, sandbagging operations, traffic barricades and signage for evacuations, etc.

ICS Forms 201, 202, 214 and 215a may be used during planning for such an incident.

Respond

During a weather-related disaster declaration, typical responses become more difficult and time consuming. Therefore, prioritization of requests becomes critical. It is important that public safety answering points be capable of providing medical instructions to callers.

A mass casualty situation during a weather-related disaster will be very challenging for the first EMS unit on scene. Depending on road conditions, a single EMS unit may need to care for many patients for a significant period of time while awaiting additional units. As with all MCIs, media attention and concerned family members are very likely. Therefore, a PIO should be appointed.

Recover

Recovery from an event such as this depends primarily on the damage caused. Recovery may be as simple as normal cleaning and restocking of units, or it may take months or years for a community to fully recover when critical infrastructure is damaged or destroyed.

Careful tracking of expenses is necessary for an EMS agency to have any possibility of receiving disaster assistance funds.

Large College Sporting Event

Large college sporting events are similar to smaller sporting events, with an added layer of complexity and visibility. Most of the same considerations apply, with a few additions.

Prepare

Preparing for a large college sporting event such as a football or basketball game begins with collecting information such as:

- requesting agency, point of contact, and contact information for follow-up;
- financial compensation information if applicable;
- location of event(s) including intended staging location of ambulance and crew, ingress and egress routes from event;
- contact information for the teams athletic trainer/sports medicine personnel;
- contact information for any security or event personnel involved; and
- anticipated/historical attendance numbers, issues.

When this information has been obtained, a risk assessment should be performed (if one has not already been done for this type of event). Contact should be made with any other involved medical personnel to coordinate operations:

- Athletic trainers.
    - Athletic trainers may be able to assist with injured players.
    - Athletic trainers may be trained in CPR/AED and are likely to be first on scene if a player collapses.
- Sports medicine staff.
    - Sports medicine staff will be able to assist with injured players.
    - Sports medicine staff should be trained in CPR/AED and are likely to arrive before EMS.
- Security staff.
    - Security staff may have CPR/AED training and should know where AEDs are located at the event. Security staff will be helpful in locating or moving ill or injured spectators.
    - Security staff will also be able to help in guiding additional medical resources to the incident.
- Fire department or EMS agency (if different from your own) that has jurisdiction over the location of the event.
    - If your agency does not have jurisdiction, the agency with jurisdiction may choose to respond and assume control of any incident that occurs.

Ten Largest U.S. Stadiums By Seating Capacity–College				
Stadium	Team	City	State	Seats
Michigan Stadium	University of Michigan	Ann Arbor	MI	109,901
Beaver Stadium	Penn State University	University Park	PA	107,282
Neyland Stadium	University of Tennessee	Knoxville	TN	102,455
Ohio Stadium	Ohio State University	Columbus	OH	102,329
Bryant-Denny Stadium	University of Alabama	Tuscaloosa	AL	101,821
Texas Memorial Stadium	University of Texas	Austin	TX	100,119
Los Angeles Memorial Coliseum	University of Southern CA	Los Angeles	CA	93,607
Sanford Stadium	University of Georgia	Athens	GA	92,746
Rose Bowl	University of CA Los Angeles	Pasadena	CA	92,542
Tiger Stadium	Louisiana State University	Baton Rouge	LA	92,400

Ten Largest U.S. Stadiums By Seating Capacity–Professional				
Stadium	Team	City	State	Seats
FedEx Field	Washington Redskins	Landover	MD	91,704
New Meadowlands Stadium	NY Giants/Jets	East Rutherford	NJ	82,566
Cowboys Stadium	Dallas Cowboys	Arlington	TX	80,000
Arrowhead Stadium	Kansas City Chiefs	Kansas City	MO	79,101
EverBank Field	Jacksonville Jaguars	Jacksonville	FL	76,876
Invesco Field at Mile High	Denver Broncos	Denver	CO	76,125
Sun Life Stadium	Miami Dolphins	Miami Gardens	FL	74,916
Ralph Wilson Stadium	Buffalo Bills	Orchard Park	NY	73,967
Bank of America Stadium	Carolina Panthers	Charlotte	NC	73,298
Cleveland Browns Stadium	Cleveland Browns	Cleveland	OH	73,200

Additional Resources:
- National Athletic Trainers' Association.
- Your State's Athletic Trainers' Association.
- American Medical Society for Sports Medicine.
- American College of Sports Medicine.
- National Academy of Sports Medicine.
- American Orthopedic Society for Sports Medicine.
- American Medical Athletic Association.
- Local volunteer groups and county/local medical society.

Forms:
- ICS Forms 202, 204, 205, and 206 will likely be needed during planning for an event such as this.
- ICS Forms 207 (Incident Organization Chart) and 214 may be required as well.

Respond

Responding to an emergency at any spectator sport will become a high-visibility event. Inevitably, photos and video of the responding personnel will be available on the internet within minutes of the incident occurring. If an event occurs in the stands, parking lot, or other areas, security and other event personnel might not be aware of the emergency. This is where the EMS planning related to collection of contact information will become useful. Communication personnel can use the contact information to notify event staff as well as direct them to acquire an AED or other equipment if applicable.

If issues arose during the response or patient treatment that have attracted the attention of conventional or social media, a PIO needs to be appointed for the incident and active management of the situation should begin.

Recover

Recovery from this type of event should not be overly complex. Recovery will likely be limited to cleaning and restocking equipment according to SOPs. In instances involving emotionally charged situations, such as unsuccessful resuscitation of a child, debriefing or CISM may be indicated.

If the incident involved numerous units or lasted several hours, demobilization procedures should be followed and recorded on ICS Form 221 to ensure that mutual aid and other resources are properly accounted for and returned to service.

Political Assembly

Political assemblies or rallies are often emotionally charged events involving groups with diametrically opposed viewpoints. Significant potential for conflict exists. Planning for political events will primarily be handled by law enforcement or security services.

Most political events involve significant intelligence gathering and coordination. Security services and law enforcement personnel will frequently be aware of and involved in discussions concerning sensitive information, which if available publicly, could endanger lives and safety. A basic premise of information security is to share information only with those that absolutely need to have access to the information. This means that if a piece of information is relevant to a particular discipline, then that information should be shared, but if the information will not change how EMS responds to or plans for an event, then there is no need to share that information. EMS planners may feel put-off by being excluded from certain meetings and planning activities, but this is a normal part of information security and should not be taken personally.

If EMS planners want law enforcement and security services to include them in their planning process, they must learn and respect the rules of information security. EMS planners that allow information to leak across their organization or from their organization to the public are not only demonstrating that they cannot be trusted with sensitive information, they are also endangering lives and safety.

Prepare

Information gathering may be more difficult or compressed chronologically due to information security concerns. Close coordination with the following groups or individuals will help ensure that EMS planners are properly informed and prepared for all likely scenarios.

- lead law enforcement agency;
- involved political officials;
- event organizers/planners;
- press agencies covering the event;
- State information fusion center;
- emergency management officials;
- public health department;
- representatives from area hospitals;
- EMAC (See Annex III for additional information);
- department of public works;
- State police;
- national disaster medical system; and
- national guard.

Additional Resources:
- National Tactical Officers Association.
- U.S. Secret Service.

Forms:
ICS Forms 201, 202, 203, 205, 206, 215a and 226 (Individual Performance Rating) may all be required during event planning. ICS Forms 200, 204, 214 and 215 are likely to be used during the actual event.

Respond
Credentialing and entry control are critical parts of high-security events such as political assemblies. This means that responding units may have their entry into certain areas delayed if proper security procedures are not followed before and during these types of events. Mass casualty events occurring within or as a result of political assemblies may require greater emphasis on personnel accountability and patient/victim segregation and control. Any incident that could be the result of hostile action will require that law enforcement identify and question each patient/victim. Normally, permitting those with minor or no injuries to leave the scene is an effective way to reduce the patient load, but law enforcement will likely detain and question these individuals. This often results in either the individual or law enforcement requesting that EMS personnel evaluate or treat these victims. Therefore, planning considerations should include more substantial staffing and focus on the green or minor patient treatment area.

Responders should be prepared to treat multiple patients exposed to riot control agents. Responders should be prepared to protect themselves from these agents as well as provide effective mass decontamination. Responders should keep careful records of costs incurred for potential future reimbursement.

Demobilization from large incidents within these events may require use of ICS Form 221.

Auto Racing/Competition

Automobile racing and other forms of automotive competition often involve very high speeds and significant potential for injury to competitors and spectators alike. Some modern speedways are designed to prevent out of control vehicles from endangering spectators, but even at these venues, there are numerous pit crew and other event personnel that are not fully protected by these barricades. Therefore, the potential for mass casualties with very significant injuries exists.

Automobile competition encompasses a wide range of different events and vehicles. From high speed NASCAR events to low speed but high-energy truck pulls to off road racing, each type of event offers unique challenges to EMS planners.

Prepare
As with all planning, gather critical background information:

- point of contact with event personnel;
- point of contact with event security personnel;
- expected attendance;
- details about safety equipment unique to event vehicles such as helmets, fuel and electrical cut-offs, or HANS (Head And Neck Support) system devices;
- details about course access procedures, ingress and egress routes; and
- details about medical aid stations, if applicable.

When this information has been obtained, a very brief risk assessment should be performed (if one has not already been done for this type of event). Contact should be made with any other involved personnel to coordinate operations:

- Medical aid station personnel (if not from your service).
  - Coordinate staffing and stocking of medical supplies and equipment.
- Rescue technicians responsible for extrication of drivers from vehicles.
  - Coordinate precisely where areas of responsibility lie, such as provision of cervical immobilization equipment or other medical equipment.
- Fire suppression personnel.
  - Coordinate who is responsible for clearing EMS personnel to approach after a crash.
  - Define hot, warm, and cold zones during extrication process.
- Any other medical personnel involved.
  - Course/Event physicians.
  - Helicopter pilots and personnel.
- Off-road vehicle clubs.
  - For off-road vehicle races, access to the course can be extremely difficult. Off-road clubs may be able to provide drivers and vehicles to transport EMS personnel out onto the course.

- Amateur radio clubs.
  - If radio coverage is an issue on a larger course, amateur radio clubs may be able to provide supplemental, long-range communication capabilities to rescue personnel.

Respond

EMS personnel must exercise extreme caution when operating on or near vehicle race tracks. Defined safety procedures must be followed to ensure that drivers on the course are notified and reduce speed prior to any personnel attempting to enter the area. EMS personnel must follow direction from course officials on when to ingress or egress an area. Failure to follow directions could result in injuries not only to EMS personnel but also could result in crashes and other injuries.

A mass casualty situation during this type of event could involve numerous hazards and significant mechanism of injury. Careful coordination between involved agencies will be necessary to effectively manage this type of event.

ICS Form 206 is likely the only ICS Form that EMS personnel may be responsible for during this type of event. During the event, ICS Form 214 may be requested from medical personnel. Use caution when completing this form as it should not include any Health Insurance Portability and Accountability Act (HIPAA) protected information.

Recover

No unique recovery actions are likely. Due to media coverage, EMS public relations staff may wish to become involved. Protracted or complicated events may require the use of ICS Form 221.

Cancer Walk

These types of events usually involve thousands of participants walking from point to point during the day and sleeping, eating, and showering in temporary facilities constructed for their use. These events usually involve significant numbers of heat and other types of injuries. EMS resources may be requested to respond anywhere along a 20 mile route or they may be requested to respond to the temporary "tent city" erected to support the participants and staff. These events are dynamic and logistically complex. Careful coordination with event organizers will be necessary to ensure EMS resources are in the right places at the right time, in sufficient quantity.

These types of events create complex coordination issues due to their geographic scope. Simultaneously, the tent city may be in one jurisdiction, many of the participants may be in another jurisdiction, and a few participants may even be in a third jurisdiction. Careful coordination is necessary to ensure that all portions of the event are appropriately covered.

Due to the fact that these events are rarely held in the same location year after year, it may be difficult for an EMS agency to gain experience covering this type of event. This means that previous operational plans, participant numbers, and response histories for the event may need to be acquired from other agencies in order to form a clear picture of what to expect.

Prepare

This type of event will require careful coordination with the following groups or individuals:

- The event organizers.
  - Event organizers may be contracting for medical services, or the event operations management firm may be in charge of this.
  - Financial compensation.
- The event operations management company.
  - Clearly define who has authority for coordinating EMS response and management of multiple casualty incidents.
  - Define clear roles and responsibilities for EMS response to each area of the course, to the medical aid stations on the course, and for staffing of medical aid stations.
  - Determine communication methods and channels.
- Involved public health departments.
  - Ensuring food safety and sanitation during event.
  - May be involved in staffing or inspection of medical aid stations.
- Department of public works.
  - Street closures, movable barricades, temporary signage, etc.
- All fire, police, and EMS agencies that will be impacted or involved in the event.
  - Critical to define areas of responsibility.
  - There may be jurisdiction issues if the event management company wants a single EMS agency to oversee the entire event, when the event moves outside that agencies jurisdiction.

- Representatives from impacted hospitals.
  - Potential for increased load.
  - Medical aid stations may be staffed by hospital nurses or physicians, affecting available staff on days of the event.
- Aeromedical.
  - If portions of the course are significant distance from level one or level two trauma centers, consider scouting potential helicopter landing zones along those sections of the course.

Although the event operations management firm may choose to use ICS forms for documenting the event operations plan, EMS planners will likely only be called upon to complete a 206 (Medical Plan). Alternatively, the event 206 may be prepared by medical aid station or other personnel.

Respond

Although a lead EMS agency contracted by the event management firm may be able to gain permission to respond to individual participants within another agency's jurisdiction during the event, it is highly unlikely that the same EMS agency will permit an outside agency to run a high-visibility MCI that occurs within their jurisdiction. This has the potential to create enormous command and control issues during a mass care incident. These issues must be anticipated and solutions agreed-upon by all involved.

Some areas of a course may be difficult to access by conventional ambulance, so alternative response vehicles such as bikes, motorcycles, or golf carts may be required.

It is important to notify event operation personnel of emergencies at the event that are called into 9-1-1. Operations personnel may not be immediately aware of these events but may have event personnel that can help locate callers or provide first aid or CPR while awaiting EMS arrival.

Recover

Recovery from an MCI should require only minimal documentation and demobilization compared to normal restocking, cleaning, and documentation procedures. As with most mass casualty incidents, significant media attention is likely, and therefore a public relations representative should be appointed.

Reimbursement for expenses during an incident might be obtainable from the event operations management firm, but careful records will be critical as multiple agencies may attempt to recover expenses for same or similar services.

For extremely protracted or involved incidents, an ICS Form 221 may be needed.

This page was intentionally left blank.

SECTION III: Case Studies in Mass Incident Deployment

Case 1: 2010 Bus Crash in Hartford, CT

Introduction
This case illustrates the need for solid local mutual aid agreements and protocols between Emergency Medical Services (EMS) agencies. EMS personnel from four different agencies were required to adequately manage this incident. Planning and the use of agency-to-agency mutual aid agreements set the stage for successful management of the incident.

Incident Summary
On Saturday, January 9, 2010, a school bus from the Greater Hartford Academy of Math and Science departed from Hartford, CT, with 16 students and a teacher aboard to bring students to a high school. A collision occurred between the bus and a Volvo station wagon as they were traveling on Interstate 84, causing the bus to go off the highway and proceed down an embankment. The bus then came to rest approximately 50 feet below the roadway. The students and the teacher on the bus suffered multiple injuries. A passer-by called 9-1-1.

Unified Command (UC) was established by the Hartford Fire Department (HFD). The first responding Chief Officer established command, then took over the Operations Section Chief role once the second responding Chief Officer was briefed and took command of the fire response. The first responding EMS supervisor assumed command of the EMS response and assigned personnel to triage and transport the patients. After an extensive rescue operation by the HFD, 17 patients were transported to local hospitals by several private EMS agencies.

Key Response Partners
Fire Agencies (Emergency Support Function (ESF)-4)
Local Fire Department–Hartford Fire Department

EMS Agencies (ESF-8)
Local EMS Agency–AETNA

Local EMS Agency–AMR-Hartford

Regional Mutual Aid EMS Agency–AMR-Waterbury

Regional Mutual Aid EMS Agency–ASM

Hospitals (ESF-8)
Saint Francis Hospital

Hartford Hospital

Connecticut Children's Medical Center

John Dempsey Hospital

Law Enforcement Agencies (ESF-13)
State Police–Connecticut State Police

Local Police–Hartford Police Department

EMS Mass Incident Deployment Pearls

Fire Agency Role in Patient Triage
HFD established UC at the scene of this incident. Facing a complex rescue and extrication operation, the bulk of HFD resources were focused on patient access. During that critical step, HFD supplied triage tags to responding EMS resources to facilitate the patient triage process in addition to providing personnel to directly triage patients in cooperation with EMS resources.

EMS Mutual Aid (Local and Regional)
The EMS response to this incident was achieved through the activation of regional agency-to-agency mutual aid agreements. The first-arriving agency, AETNA, assumed command of EMS operations and requested 11 additional ambulances. Additional resources included five ambulances from AMR (Hartford), three ambulances from AMR (Waterbury), and three ambulances from ASM.

In the After Action Report (AAR) of this incident, there was some confusion as to the precise position the EMS supervisor occupied in the Incident Command System (ICS). EMS representative to the UC was one option, while EMS Branch Director was the other. Agencies should ensure that they establish a clear position in the ICS for EMS functions in coordination with response partners.

Law Enforcement Role in Patient Tracking and Flow
In this incident, the Connecticut State Police have statutory responsibility for the overall management of interstate highway mishaps in Connecticut. As part of this responsibility, the patient tracking element normally located in ESF-8 was integrated with the ESF-13 function. This element was operationalized through the deployment of State troopers to the hospitals to assist with management of patient flow in addition to communication with transporting EMS resources at the scene to ensure a complete count of patients.

Reference
- City of Hartford After Action Report. *Motor Vehicle/Bus Accident I84 Westbound,* January 2010.

Case 2: 2005 F3 Tornado in Marshall County, KY

Introduction

This case demonstrates how the number of casualties does not always dictate the scope and complexity of the EMS response. EMS personnel from four agencies worked together to treat and transport 21 patients in Marshall County, KY, during a rash of tornados that impacted a four county region and extended into neighboring States. Although the initial response was local in nature, it quickly evolved to include response partners at regional, statewide, and Federal levels.

Incident Summary

An F3 tornado struck portions of Marshall County, KY, on Tuesday, November 15, 2005, at approximately 2:15 p.m. The tornado caused minimal damage in the southwest corner of the county. The tornado then cut a path of destruction for 10.8 miles toward the northeast. The width of the tornado was 475 to 500 yards in some locations. Over 120 residences were damaged, with 19 being totally destroyed. There were 113 camper trailers at a local campground and only 2 were left salvageable. There was 1 fatality at a mobile home park and over 20 individuals were injured as a result of the event.

The ensuing response required a true multidisciplinary approach. Initial search and rescue efforts were conducted by county volunteer fire agencies with support from Marshall County Rescue Squad. The EMS command was established as part of the countywide unified command by Marshall County EMS personnel. The coordinated mutual aid response was organized through the Marshall County Emergency Operations Center (EOC). Initial actions were focused on providing rescue operations, emergency medical operations, and management of mass shelter operations.

Key Response Partners

Transportation Agencies (ESF-1)

Kentucky Department of Transportation

Marshall County Road Department

Graves County Road Department

Livingston County Road Department

Communications Agencies (ESF-2)

Marshall County Amateur Radio Association

Marshall County 911

Public Works and Engineering Agencies (ESF-3)

West Kentucky Rural Telephone and Technology

West Kentucky Rural Electric

Fire Agencies (ESF-4)

Eleven Marshall County Volunteer Fire Departments

Emergency Management Agencies (ESF-5)

Kentucky Division of Emergency Management

Marshall County Emergency Management

Mass Care, Emergency Assistance Agencies (ESF-6)

Lakeland Red Cross

Mt. Carmel Methodist Church

Emergency Medical Services Agencies (ESF-8)

Marshall County EMS

Mercy Regional EMS

Livingston County EMS

Calloway County EMS

Public Health Agencies (ESF-8)

Kentucky Department of Health

Marshall County Department of Health

Hospitals (ESF-8)

Marshall County Hospital

Search and Rescue Agency (ESF-9)

Marshall County Rescue Squad

Law Enforcement Agencies (ESF-13)

U.S. Coast Guard

Kentucky National Guard

Kentucky State Police

Kentucky Vehicle Enforcement

Marshall County Sheriff's Office

Benton Police Department

EMS Mass Incident Deployment Pearls
Overall Incident Complexity

This incident resulted in the disruption of public infrastructure including power outages, numerous blocked roadways, and disruption in phone services. Responders mobilized local, regional, and State resources in an organized and progressive manner. EMS operational goals and objectives centered on supporting rescue operations to locate and extricate persons trapped in damaged structures, provision of emergency medical services, and maintaining essential public services. Planning the integration of EMS operations into the overall disaster response through coordination and structured agreements with the primary agencies responsible for managing each Emergency Support Function that could be brought in to play in an incident such as this enhances the efficiency, safety, and effectiveness of the response.

Use of Satellite Phones

Satellite phones and computers provided by West Kentucky Rural Telephone in addition to satellite phones equipped on the Marshall County Mobile Command Post were used to coordinate with Marshall County Emergency Management and other response partners. The use of satellite phones is a viable alternative to cellular communications in the event of network overload or outage. If satellite technology is included in the communications plan within the jurisdiction, it is important to ensure that end user personnel are familiar with the operation, limitations, and utility of the specific devices they will be using during a deployment.

References

- NOAA Forecast Office Paducha, KY. *Damage Survey Results for Marshall County Kentucky*, November 15, 2005.

- Marshall County Emergency Management. *After Action Report*, December 12, 2005.

Case 3: 2010 Veterans Administration Hospital Evacuation, Lebanon, PA

Introduction

This incident demonstrates the importance of regional coordination of EMS transport assets. Pennsylvania uses a regional model to coordinate EMS response to major incidents. Though this was primarily a weather-related evacuation under controlled conditions, the initial responding agency recognized the need for regional asset activation early on. The Lebanon County Emergency Management Agency managed the requests for additional assets, and regional task force leadership ensured effective integration of assets into the onscene ICS.

Incident Summary

In July 2010, south central Pennsylvania was in the midst of a heat wave. Temperatures were consistently above 90 degrees. On July 21, 2010, a day where the heat index was 104 degrees, the Lebanon Pennsylvania Veterans Administration Medical Center experienced an environmental emergency at their facility. Temperatures in the hospital had become elevated due to problems with the air conditioning system in the hospital. Due to concerns about patient safety, hospital administration made the decision to evacuate the facility. The resulting EMS response lasted 26 hours during which 50 ambulances and wheelchair vans and 150 personnel were used to move 79 patients to several receiving facilities across two States.

Key Response Partners

Transportation Agencies (ESF-1)

Northern Lancaster County Transport

Lebanon Transit

Emergency Management Agencies (ESF-5)

Lancaster County Emergency Management Agency

Lebanon County Emergency Management Agency

Emergency Medical Services Agencies (ESF-8)

Central Medical Ambulance

Cumberland Goodwill EMS

Duncannon EMS

First Aid and Safety Patrol

Life Team EMS

Manheim Township EMS

Northwest EMS

SCTF EMS Task Force 38 (Dauphin/Lebanon)

SCTF EMS Task Force 36 (Lancaster)

SCTF EMS Task Force 67 (York)

SCTF EMS Task Force 21 (Cumberland/Perry)

Emergency Medical Services Agencies (ESF-8) (continued)

South Central EMS

Susquehanna Township EMS

Susquehanna Valley EMS

Upper Dauphin County EMS

Warwick Community Ambulance

West Shore EMS

White Rose Ambulance

Hospitals (ESF-8)

Altoona Veterans Administration Medical Center

Coatesville Veterans Medical Center

Good Samaritan Hospital, Lebanon

Heart of Lancaster Medical Center, Lancaster

Holy Spirit Hospital, Camp Hill

Horsham Clinic

Lancaster Hospice

Lebanon Veterans Administration Medical Center

Manor Care, York

Penn State Milton S. Hershey Medical Center

Philadelphia Veterans Medical Center

Philhaven

Reading Hospital

Wilmington (DE) Veterans Administration Medical Center

Wilkes-Barre Veterans Medical Center

EMS Mass Incident Deployment Pearls
Regional Structure for Mass Incident Response

This incident made extensive use of regional EMS response teams. The South Central Task Force (SCTF) is one of nine regional counter-terrorism task forces in Pennsylvania. SCTF encompasses an 8-county region, covering an area of approximately 5,200 square miles and a population of over 1.7 million. Within the south central region, there are 312 municipalities. Over 90 percent of fire/rescue organizations are volunteer-based, including the hazardous materials and Urban Search and Rescue (US&R)/technical rescue units. There are 326 fire departments, 143 police departments, and 135 ambulance services in the region. The efforts used to catalog and plan deployment of those resources proved invaluable during this incident.

Participation in regional teams is voluntary. Funding for the program comes from Federal grants. SCTF provides a common framework to coordinate operations, communications, and protocols during a mass incident. In this case, teams activated through this mechanism arrived at the incident with transport capable ambulances and personnel. The teams did not bring the equipment and Incident Command Trailers assigned to each team due to the nature of the incident. However, each task force has organic ICS capability. Organizing EMS assets into regional task force elements provides an organized means to deploy assets during an emergency.

References

- Noll, G. "Regional Response to All-Hazards Events: A Commonwealth Perspective." *Commonwealth*, Vol. 15-3, May 2009.

- South Central Task Force. *Lebanon (PA) Veterans Administration Medical Center Evacuation-EMS Operations After Action Report/Improvement Plan*, November 2010.

Case 4: 2008 Imperial Sugar Dixie Crystal Plant Fire, Port Wentworth, GA

Introduction

This incident occurred in a predominantly rural area in South Georgia. The explosion and fire resulted in 14 fatalities and triggered EMS and fire response stretching across 12 counties. The response was an exercise in managed chaos in which incident managers throughout the ICS were challenged with communication, logistics, finances, and personnel accountability problems that stretched existing plans to the limit.

Incident Summary

At approximately 7:20 p.m. Thursday, February 7, 2008, a dust initiated explosion and fire occurred at the 872,000 square foot Imperial Sugar Dixie Crystal Plant in Port Wentworth, GA. The explosion destroyed three large reinforced concrete sugar elevators and several buildings. The resulting fire spread throughout the majority of the plant resulting in concentrated pools of molten burning sugar. At the time of the incident there were 121 employees and contractors. There were 36 people injured and transported to Memorial hospital; of those, 14 were non-life-threatening injuries. Nineteen victims were transported to the Augusta Burn Center. Over the following week, search efforts recovered the remains of eight missing workers from the debris. Additional fatalities were recorded as patients succumbed to their injuries. The final (14th) fatality occurred 200 days following the event.

This incident stimulated political debate at the State and Federal level culminating in legislation that is aimed at preventing similar incidents.

Key Response Partners

Over 200 agencies participated in this incident. The following is a sampling identified in the AAR from the incident.

Fire and EMS Agencies (ESF-4) (ESF-8)

Ft. Oglethorpe Fire Department

Garden City Fire Department

Port Wentworth Fire Department

Pooler Fire Department

Thunderbolt Fire Department

Savannah Fire Department

Savannah Chatham Metropolitan Police

Bloomingdale Fire Department

Emergency Management Agencies (ESF-5)

Chatham County Emergency Management Agency (CEMA)

Georgia Emergency Management Agency (GEMA)

Mass Care, Emergency Assistance Agencies (ESF-6)

Salvation Army

Savannah Chapter of American Red Cross

Low Country Health District, South Carolina

Search and Rescue (ESF-9)

Georgia Search and Rescue Team (GSAR)

Georgia Department of Corrections Canine Teams

Georgia Body Recovery Team

Hospitals (ESF-8)

Candler Hospital

Memorial Hospital

St. Joseph's Hospital

Joseph M. Still Burn Center, Augusta, GA

EMS Mass Incident Deployment Pearls
Effective Triage to Specialty Care Centers

The triage process identified 19 patients with significant burns that required specialty care. Patients were triaged, and then transported to Memorial Hospital for stabilizing care. In the midst of a complex rescue, paramedics from the Savannah Fire Department and other agencies proactively identified patients that would require specialty transport and communicated up through the ICS to ensure that appropriate air medical and ground transport assets were allocated to transport the patients to the Joseph M. Still Burn Center in Augusta. Though the AAR identifies several issues with the distribution of patients, particularly the decision to not send patients to St. Joseph Hospital at all, and send just seven patients to Candler Hospital, the overall triage system in this event correctly identified critical burn patients that required advanced specialized care and ensured that they were transported to a facility with adequate landing facilities that would accommodate air medical evacuation assets. This identification expedited the process of acquiring specialty care and ultimately saved lives.

Coordination with Federal Aviation Administration

The Incident Commander (IC) in cooperation with county and State emergency management agencies requested that the Federal Aviation Administration (FAA) institute Temporary Flight Restrictions (TFR) that ensured that only emergency flights would be authorized in the airspace surrounding the incident. When requested, the FAA immediately instituted the requested flight restrictions. Exceptions to the TFR were coordinated through the County Emergency Management Agency. EMS and incident planners should consider working with emergency managers to institute flight restrictions for incidents where there will be significant traffic due to the use of air medical assets, fire suppression assets, or aerial surveillance and survey platforms.

Personnel Safety: Consultation with Structural Engineer

Due to the depth of the catalog of assets available to emergency managers at this incident, when it was discovered that consultation with a structural engineer was needed to provide the safest possible operating environment for rescue and triage personnel, the County Emergency Management Agency was able to locate and mobilize a structural engineer within an hour of requesting the asset. Planners should identify structural engineers within their jurisdiction with the expertise and willingness to assist in an emergency situation, then equip and train those engineers to ensure a proper state of readiness to respond to an emergency.

Reference

- Chatham Emergency Management Agency. *After Action Report: Imperial Sugar Dixie Crystal Plant*, April 2008.

Case 5: 2006 Woodward Dream Cruise, Berkley, MI

Introduction

This annual event emphasizes the importance of local coordination for multijurisdictional events. EMS is provided for this event via a combination of traditional fire based systems, private ambulance services, and public safety departments. Public safety departments fulfill law enforcement, fire, and EMS roles within their local jurisdiction. Planning is accomplished through a multidisciplinary, multiagency group representing the full spectrum of public safety and public health services.

Incident Summary

The Woodward Dream Cruise is the world's largest one-day automotive event, drawing about 1.5 million people and 40,000 classic cars. This population is distributed along a 14 mile stretch of road running from the city of Detroit to the City of Pontiac in southeast Michigan. The event involves participants driving a circuit, and engaging in demonstrations that highlight the capability of muscle cars and other high performance vehicles. The event is scheduled to occur on a single day, but in reality covers a three day operational period, resulting in multiple planning and logistical challenges for EMS planners. EMS volume results from exacerbation of chronic illnesses among the spectators, and minor traumatic injuries. In 2006, the event resulted in over 93 EMS transports to local hospitals and 328 patient contacts from EMS assets over a 24-hour operational period.

Key Response Partners

Communications (ESF-2)

Oakland County ARES/RACES

Fire Agencies (ESF-4)

Berkley Public Safety Department

Birmingham Fire Department

Bloomfield Hills Public Safety

Bloomfield Township Fire Department

Detroit Fire Department

Ferndale Fire Department

Huntington Woods Public Safety Department

Pontiac Fire Department

Royal Oak Fire Department

Emergency Management Agencies (ESF-5)

Oakland County Emergency Management

Public Health Agencies (ESF-8)

Oakland County Public Health

Emergency Medical Services Agencies (ESF-8)

Alliance Mobile Health

Berkley Public Safety

Birmingham Fire Department EMS

Bloomfield Hills Public Safety

Bloomfield Township Fire Department

Detroit Fire Department EMS

Ferndale Fire Department EMS

Huntington Woods Public Safety

Pontiac Fire Department EMS

Royal Oak Fire Department EMS

Star EMS

Hospitals (ESF-8)

Beaumont Hospital Royal Oak

Doctors Hospital Pontiac

Pontiac Osteopathic Hospital

Providence Hospital Southfield

St. Joseph Medical Center

Law Enforcement (ESF-13)

Berkley Public Safety

Birmingham Police Department

Bloomfield Hills Public Safety

Bloomfield Township Police Department

Detroit Police Department

Ferndale Police Department

Huntington Woods Public Safety

Oakland County Sheriff Department

Pleasant Ridge Police Department

Michigan State Police

Law Enforcement (ESF-13) (Continued)

Pontiac Police Department

Royal Oak Police Department

Wayne County Sheriff Department

EMS Mass Incident Deployment Pearls
Coordination Between Multiple Jurisdictions and Service Models

Oakland County, MI, provides EMS service via several models. During usual operations, EMS agencies of different types do not ordinarily interact. This event stimulates interaction between the various delivery models in the county, and takes advantage of formal mutual aid agreements between agencies. Due to traffic congestion, EMS agencies respond across jurisdictions and operate in a cooperative manner throughout the operational period. In addition, special event assets such as bike teams, and nontraditional EMS units such as Gators and golf carts provide first response services across jurisdictions. Emergency planners that have disparate EMS service models within their jurisdiction should collaborate to ensure seamless operational protocols in the event of a planned or unplanned mass incident.

Communications in a Multijurisdictional Incident

Following the terrorist attacks of September 11, 2001, Oakland County made the decision to implement a countywide Internet Protocol (IP) based radio system titled Oakland County Wireless Integrated Network (OakWIN). This system has the capability to coordinate communications across the entire public safety spectrum including the use of common talk groups and talk paths that enable seamless communication across political jurisdictions. The system is designed to support live patching so that users in one talk group can be integrated into another talk group as needed. This facilitates communication between response entities across disciplines. Communications is one of the most frequently cited areas of concern in incident after action reviews. This system addresses many of those concerns and lessons learned from the implementation of this system could be useful to emergency planners.

References

- OCMCA. *After Action Review: EMS at Woodward Dream Cruise*, November 2006.
- CLEMIS. *OAKWIN User Manual*, October 2005.

Case 6: 2010 Ironman Triathlon Event, St. George, UT

Introduction

Ironman St. George is a 140.6 mile triathlon (swim/bike/run) on the World Triathlon Corporation Ironman racing circuit. Casualties are common due to temperature and the sheer difficulty of the bike and run courses. For the 2010 event, Utah Department of Health EMS Strike Team and Regional Strike Team established a 100 bed medical station at the swim location.

Incident Summary

The Utah Department of Health, EMS Strike Team and Regional Strike Team (Southwest Regional Response Team) supported the Ford Ironman St. George event, May 1, 2010. The Ironman event consisted of athletic participation in three sequential stages—the swim (2.4 mile), bike (112 mile), and run (26.2 mile) event. There are time cutoffs to complete each stage with an overall time not to exceed 17 hours. In this event 1,915 athletes started the race.

The Strike Teams' role in the event was to establish four 25 bed BLU-MED tents at the swim venue to ensure immediate access to care in the event of an emergency. Due to the low water temperature of 59 degrees, and the extended period of immersion, 60 athletes presented to the tent with hypothermia. Advanced treatment was required for 38 athletes who were so ill, they were not permitted to continue the race. Due to the interventions of the Strike Teams, no athletes required transportation to the hospital.

Key Response Partners

Some event locations were staffed by Utah Homeland Security, local law enforcement, EMS, and fire departments not specifically enumerated in the AAR.

Fire Agencies (ESF-4)

Hurricane Fire Department

Emergency Medical Services Agencies (ESF-8)

Hurricane Fire Department

Utah Department of Health, Bureau of Emergency Medical Service

Southwest Regional Response Team

Public Health Agencies (ESF-8)

Southwest Utah Public Health Department

Hospitals (ESF-8)

Dixie Regional Medical Center

Salt Lake City Veteran Affairs Medical Center (VA)

External Affairs (ESF-15)

World Triathlon Association

Ford Ironman St. George Planning Committee

EMS Mass Incident Deployment Pearls
Prevention of Unnecessary Ambulance Transports

The presence of the Strike Teams and associated temporary medical facility prevented transfer of patients to the hospital for simple hypothermia. This resulted in improved efficiency for the entire medical operation at the event. Ambulances were not needed to move patients that essentially needed to be rewarmed. Treating patients that are safe to keep at the event site in lieu of transport also preserves emergency room (ER) capacity for more serious events should they occur.

Use of Special Events as Opportunity to Exercise Capabilities

In addition to the primary provision of medical care, the Utah Department of Health Strike Team used the Ironman St. George event as an opportunity to exercise their mobilization and demobilization procedures, use of the ICS, and communications strategies under real world conditions. Planners should seek opportunities to exercise capabilities at preplanned special events when appropriate.

Reference
- Utah Department of Public Health. *Ford Ironman St. George Triathlon*, May 2010.

Case 7: 2004 Democratic National Convention, Boston, MA

Introduction

The 2004 Democratic National Convention (DNC) required the planning and execution of medical operations within a complex security environment. Boston Emergency Medical Services (Boston EMS) developed a Medical Consequence Management Plan that serves as a model for the medical management of National Special Security Events to this day. Though elements of the plan are not suitable for wide dissemination, the following planning pearls are useful for the implementation of medical plans at virtually any larger venue.

Incident Summary

The 2004 DNC was designated a National Special Security Event (NSSE) by the Department of Homeland Security (DHS). The U.S. Secret Service (USSS), the Federal Bureau of Investigation (FBI), and the Federal Emergency Management Agency (FEMA) were responsible for interagency incident management coordination during the event. The USSS designated Boston EMS the lead agency for health and medical services related to the Convention. Boston EMS Chief Richard Serino was appointed to the Executive Steering Committee. As a member of the Executive Steering Committee, Chief Serino coordinated the development of the DNC Medical Consequence Management Plan.

The plan was formed through the combined effort of a panel representing 39 agencies. The resulting document was produced in hard copy and as dynamically linked Adobe PDF files for electronic dissemination. Distribution of the plan was limited to incident participants and those with a need to know. The plan served as the tactical operations plan for the event and contained clear lines of responsibility for each element of the medical community involved in the event.

In all, Boston EMS deployed to five zones spanning the scope of daily operations through protection of the secured areas immediately surrounding the event. They accomplished this through mutual aid agreements and contracts with other EMS agencies, while maintaining control of the system through the use of multiple command posts throughout the city.

Key Response Partners

Several agencies provided services to this event. For example, over 70 agencies were involved in the provision of security alone. There were agencies responsible for virtually every ESF.

Fire Agencies (ESF-4)

Boston Fire Department

Emergency Management Agencies (ESF-5)

Federal Emergency Management Agency (FEMA)

Massachusetts Emergency Management Agency

Boston Emergency Management Agency

Emergency Medical Services Agencies (ESF-8)

Boston Emergency Medical Services

American Medical Response

Armstrong Ambulance

Emergency Medical Services Agencies (ESF-8) (continued)

Eascare

Fallon Ambulance

Professional Ambulance

Hospitals (ESF-8)

Boston Medical Center

Conference of Boston Teaching Hospitals

New England Medical Center

Community Health Centers

Massachusetts General Hospital

Public Health Agencies (ESF-8)

Massachusetts Department of Public Health

Department of Health and Human Services (DHHS)

Centers for Disease Control and Prevention (CDC)

Boston Public Health Commission

Law Enforcement Agencies (ESF-13)

U.S. Secret Service (USSS)

Federal Bureau of Investigation (FBI)

Boston Police Department

Massachusetts State Police

EMS Mass Care Incident Deployment Pearls
DNC Medical Consequence Management Plan

The plan developed for this event is a model in terms of collaboration among a large network of partners across the spectrum of ESF. It encompassed the FEMA planning principles, public health methodologies, and covered every relevant element of preparation for an incident of this scope. The plan supported the needs of security planners while maintaining the need to do the greatest good for the greatest number. The plan remains a model to this day.

Preparing for and Managing Hospital Surge

The Medical Consequence Management Plan provided a template for managing a 500 patient surge due to the DNC. The plan was comprehensive in its approach. Some highlights of key provisions in the surge plan were:

- All major hospitals in Boston agreed to suspend ambulance diversion during the week of the DNC.

- Coalition Of Boston Teaching Hospitals (COBTH) agreed to reschedule most elective surgeries for the week of the DNC.

- COBTH facilities maintained a minimum of 500 free beds for the week.

- COBTH held frequent conference calls to determine total bed capacity for the City of Boston. The calls gathered information on
    - the number of intensive care and general hospitals beds available immediately; and
    - additional beds that could be available within a reasonable time.

- COBTH facilities canceled all vacation time for the week of the DNC.

- COBTH facilities developed expanded staffing plans and physician recall plans to be implemented in case of an emergency or a mass casualty incident (MCI).

- The American Red Cross (ARC) hosted a summer blood drive to increase regional capacity during the DNC. The effort increased blood supplies by 111 percent.

- The Massachusetts Ambulance Association offered to transport blood and/or organ donations if needed.

Large Scale Mutual Aid

Boston EMS negotiated agreements with ambulance service providers whereby over 200 ambulances would be available within 30 minutes or less. In addition, Boston EMS provided "mini-grants" to mutual aid ambulance providers and fire departments to purchase common medical and communications equipment. This promoted interoperability between Boston EMS, its mutual aid partners, and all public safety agencies present at the DNC.

Medical Support to Law Enforcement Activities

The Medical Consequence Management Plan called for a number of Public Order Platoons (POPs) composed of law enforcement officers, an emergency medical technician (EMT), and a paramedic to be deployed to strategic locations. The plan also called for Boston EMS bike units to work alongside Boston Police Department bike units to provide medical coverage and operational awareness for Boston EMS during the event. The plan also designated specific facilities and pathways for care for injured public safety personnel, and arrestees/detainees from the event.

Reference

- Serino, R., *Medical Consequence Management Plan for the 2004 Democratic National Convention*, LLIS.gov, 2011.

Case 8: Annual Creation Music Festival, Mount Union, PA

Introduction
Creation Festival is an annual, 4-day Christian music festival held in Mount Union, PA, at the Agape Farm. The festival is the largest Christian music festival in the country. In addition to music performed live by over 60 bands, the festival attracts leaders, speakers, and authors from multiple Christian denominations, a stage especially for children, camping, and a petting zoo. Activities also include a wide variety of Christian ceremonies including baptisms, communion, prayer group, and candle light services.

Incident Summary
This unique 4-day event is characterized by the influx of 45,000 to 108,000 people into a rural community. The lead agency for preparing for the event is the Huntingdon County Emergency Management Agency (EMA). The EMA ensures that there is a high level of coordination among the various departments and agencies used throughout the event. Of particular note, the majority of responders at the event are volunteers. This high level of coordination coupled with management of volunteer resources and solid planning has resulted in this event serving as a model for the management of planned patient surge.

Key Response Partners
Planning documents for this event name several specific agencies that span the EMS, fire, special response, law enforcement, public health, and hospital resources available to the jurisdiction.

EMS Mass Incident Response Pearls
Management of Patient Surge
There were 593 medical patients in 2011 which were processed through on site first aid services.

However, in 2005 the event generated 946 patients over the course of four days. During that operational period surge levels reached a maximum of 25 patients over a 5-minute period and 90 patients over an hour period. The key to managing this level of surge was the level and detail of planning, placement of the medical center in a strategic location with easy ingress and egress, and the thoughtful composition of volunteer medical teams. Further, the event has cross-trained medical responders at the Emergency Medical Responder (EMR) level and above that can be diverted to medical tasks should surge conditions warrant.

Medical Center Placement and Logistics
The medical center consists of two main structures placed near the main arena and adjacent to the food vendor's area. The main building is a wooden-frame facility with three treatment rooms, two bath rooms with showers, and one room with three beds for patient monitoring. Each treatment area can handle two- to three-patients. The second building is a modular trailer unit equipped with a bathroom, two treatment areas and can hold five patient beds for monitoring. The third building is the county emergency management agency's mobile medical treatment trailer. This trailer is equipped with a restroom, three treatment rooms, examination space for five patients, medical administration space, and a platform lift for wheelchair bound and immobilized patients. These facilities are air conditioned and have fresh running water, and are covered by roofs. The medical center can handle most minor suturing and fluid resuscitation cases and general complaints. Each treatment area is equipped with oxygen administration, bandaging supplies, and wound care equipment. The medical center has one AED and has a suction unit and adjunct equipment for basic airway control. During the event, there are two Advanced Life Support (ALS) units on site in which their equipment is available for use in the medical center. Patients requiring more definitive care are referred for transport or additional care.

Planning for a Mass Casualty Incident at a Mass Gathering Event

In the case of a large scale MCI (30> casualties), the EMA and festival staff employ a mass casualty response trailer stationed at a strategic location. The cafeteria, which can be converted into a care center under emergent need, can support the basic field medical care of 75 patients using the resources on site. The facility is air conditioned and has both running water and restrooms. If additional space is necessary, adjoining residential rooms can support the space for another 40 patients with limited resources.

A second mass casualty response trailer is staged off site and can be accessed within a short time of activation.

Establishing Field Triage as a Function of the Event Instead of a Reaction to an Incident

Planners instituted a field triage station to facilitate management of patients between the arena and the medical center. This station is dedicated to the first aid needs of the main crowd at the arena. An additional small-scale field triage station is placed strategically to meet the needs of attendees in the surrounding entertainment areas.

Vignette from Adam Miller, Huntingdon County Emergency Management

During an evening concert at the main stage, the crowd engaged in heavy jumping and thrashing activity due to a very popular band playing aggressive music. This type of behavior is uncommon at the main stage arena. During this event, about 30 patients presented to main stage EMS personnel over a 5-minute period with varying clinical complaints that included lacerations, serious respiratory difficulty, and traumatic injuries. Historically, the event staffed two EMS personnel on each side of the main stage. Within moments it was recognized the situation was becoming very serious and a surge force of medical personnel were summoned to establish a field triage area to the right of the main stage.

Using ICS structure, field triage, transport, and treatment personnel were placed into service. Hospitality tables and resources typically used as a picnic area were turned into patient care areas. Cots, blankets, and atmospheric control devices were brought in and implemented to ensure that patient care could be provided in the field in a safe and comfortable manner. Triage tracking tags were implemented to ensure patients were accounted for and sorted properly. Onsite ambulances began transporting patients while the backfill plan was activated to bring additional units to the site. Shuttle buses were called into a standby position to prepare to transport additional patients if necessary. All personnel with emergency medical training in any department were recalled and ordered to the field triage areas in order to assist with sorting and caring for patients. Law enforcement and public safety personnel were used to control site access and ensure the traffic corridors were secure. Within the first hour, 91 patients were triaged and treated. Of those 91 patients, only 3 required transport to local hospitals. All other patients were addressed with onsite assets.

Lessons Learned

Have a plan to establish field triage sites near stages for concert events in the outdoors.

These should be shielded from outside environments as much as possible. For summer events such as we experience, a few of the following items are very helpful to have on site at a field triage: ez up shelters, cots, blankets, misting fans, ice, towels, common emergency medical treatment and transport supplies, oxygen administration equipment, dedicated communication equipment with onsite first-aid headquarters, triage tags, lighting, privacy gowns, emergency decontamination water flow preconnects.

Ensure that all staff regardless of discipline working for any event that has training and authorization to perform EMS treatments are preidentified and credentialed.

Have a procedure and mechanisms to recall the staff quickly from any department including flexible staffing, including on duty personnel of other disciplines.

Identify the personnel that will fill the roles of treatment, triage, and transport group supervisors, before an incident occurs if possible. Better yet if this is done at the beginning of each shift.

Identify law enforcement officers to support the security of the field triage station(s) should additional security be deemed necessary.

Establish a procedure to alert your closest hospital emergency facilities as to the status and nature of your emerging event as quickly as possible.

Establish and map hot standby locations for each medical transport vehicle for each field triage station in the planning phase.

Ensure that there is a clear line of communication, and prescript a procedure, to have producers stop the event or pause, should medical (or other) conditions require the event to stop for the safety of the participants, including a pause period to establish situational awareness and conduct immediate surveillance of the originating conditions leading to the presentation of patients.

Miscellaneous Pearls

- Use of a consistent medical director has led to consistency in clinical quality and management. The current medical director has been the medical director for 23 years.

- Use of a consistent EMS Director has led to continuity in operational planning and a high level of retained planning knowledge.

- Safesite all-hazard sensors are used during the event, and monitored on site with defined response thresholds.

- The event uses back-up offsite operations, communications and staging areas and specifically designates each in the planning phase.

- The event uses sheriff department Vehicular Tactical Network (VTAC) repeaters and integrates them into the communications plan. Use of mobile repeaters greatly enhances radio coverage and system reliability.

- Multiple methods of communication with crowds are established, including use of jumbotrons and American Sign Language (ASL) interpreters.

Reference

- Miller, A. *Creation Music Festival: Chapter 1013 Special Events EMS*. Huntingdon County Emergency Management Agency, 2011.

SECTION IV: Policy Guidance for Mass Casualty Contingency Planning at Mass Gathering Events

Introduction

Mass casualty incidents (MCIs) require careful advance planning to be managed effectively. Planning for a mass gathering event (MGE) must also include some direction for an MCI occurring within the MGE. These are extremely low frequency events but have significant impact on the Emergency Medical Services (EMS) system and population as a whole when they do occur. Proper event planning and operation will greatly enhance preparedness for MCI events.

MCI and Multi Casualty Incident are terms that are used interchangeably in the literature. For this publication, MCI refers to any event that produces a volume of ill or injured victims that cannot be handled by the available responders.

Planning Considerations

STEP 1: MCI planning begins with some basic decisions concerning available time and resources. An MCI plan that must be completed in a short timeframe with severely limited resources will, of course, be less complete than a plan that can be formed over months and has sufficient resources. Planners must not only analyze resources available for an actual MCI response, but analyze the resources available for use in the planning process.

STEP 2: Planners should perform a risk analysis once resource availability questions have been answered. The risk analysis is critical to focus limited resources on hazards and threats that are both likely and severe before focusing on less likely and less severe hazards and threats.

STEP 3: When the risk analysis is completed, planners must determine which hazards and threats to plan for and which will rely on existing standard operating procedures. Planners must be realistic when making these decisions, as there is no point in preparing for an event that is completely outside the scope of on-scene resources. Expected mutual aid resources must be involved in planning as early as practical to maximize on scene coordination.

Plans for an MCI should be simple and straightforward. Experience demonstrates that the more complex a plan is, the less likely responders are to follow it. A plan that asks responders to perform very differently than their training risks irrelevance during a significant emergency.

Finally, the hazard and risk analysis should be conducted by personnel with specific training and experience in performing such studies. Common steps in performing a risk analysis include but are not limited to:

1. Create a comprehensive list of potential hazards at the event. Consult other public safety agencies, public health, military, relevant industry, businesses, as well as historical records to help form this list. ICS Form 215a (Incident Action Plan Safety and Risk Analysis) may be useful during this stage of planning.

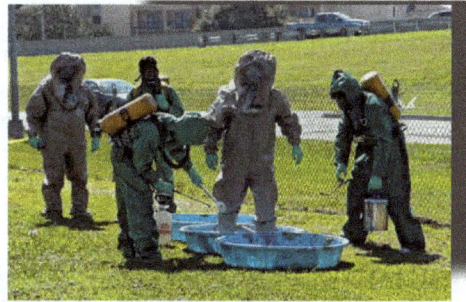

Members of an area Emergency Medical Technician team undergo training required for certification as rescue (grey suits) and decontamination (green suits) unit responders to hazardous material and toxic contamination situations.

2. For each hazard, identify vulnerable populations. Use maps to identify the geography affected, and then research the population densities for those areas. Some hazards may not be able to be isolated to particular areas, such as adverse weather. Other hazards, such as railroad tanker spills, can be easily identified by proximity to railroad tracks.

3. For each vulnerable population, assess the population's resiliency to these hazards. For instance, residents of a trailer park with no emergency shelters nearby have poor resiliency against tornadoes compared to a population living in well-constructed homes with basements. In addition, healthy adults have greater resiliency to most diseases than the elderly and children, so daycare centers and senior homes would be less resilient to a localized disease outbreak than apartments filled primarily with adults.

Create a table or chart similar to the one below.

Hazard	Vulnerable Population	Population Resilience	Relative Risk	Mitigation
Tornado	Mobile home parks	Low	Low to moderate	Early warning systems
	Outdoor venues	Moderate		
Lightning Strike	Outdoor populations	Moderate	Low	Early warning systems
Heat Injuries	Crowds	High for healthy adults	High in hot weather	Hydration stations, misting stations, etc.
	Outdoor populations	Low for elderly		
Crowd Surge or Fights	Sporting events, rock, rap, and hip-hop concerts	Moderate	Moderate	Careful layout of crowd barricades and plentiful exit routes
	Participants near stage and exits			
Structural Collapse	Participants under or on structure	Low	Low	Careful inspection of structures

Risk Mitigation

Once the risks of a particular event are known and cataloged, planners should determine how to mitigate those risks within practical constraints. For instance, if tornados are a known risk, careful weather monitoring and early warning systems may help avoid injuries due to this risk.

The largest risk during most outside events in the summer is the risk of heat injuries. This risk can be mitigated by making water and other hydration options readily available, using fans and misting systems, or providing shade with tents or other temporary structures. It is usually much more cost-effective to mitigate a risk than it is to respond to the risk once it has occurred.

Mitigation of risk should begin with high risk, high impact incidents first, then low risk high impact events, followed by low risk low impact events if time and resources permit.

Catalog Threats

Once a risk analysis is complete, analyze each hazard and determine the following:

1. What agency or group would likely command the response to the threat?

2. What would the primary and secondary objectives for each threat be?

3. Who would handle the common command positions during the response to the threat?
4. At what threshold should an emergency be declared? A disaster?
5. At what threshold should mutual aid resources be requested?
6. Who would be responsible for declaring a disaster situation? How would you contact them?

When each hazard has been analyzed, organize the responses to the questions above into an easy to understand reference document such as below.

	Law Enforcement		Fire/HazMat		Technical Rescue		Medical	
Relative Risk	High	Low	High	Low	High	Low	High	Low
Risk Analysis	Assaults	Suicide bombing, homicide	Suspicious odor investigation	Hazardous material release	None	Building collapse	Heat/Cold Injuries	Mass Food Poisoning
Command	State police		Fire department		Fire department		Public health	
Statutory Authority	Local LE or State Police		Local fire department		Regional Technical Rescue Team		Public Health Department	
Command Structure	IC with Fire/EMS branch		UC with LE, EMS, Fire		IC with EMS branch		UC with public health, hospitals, EMS	
Primary Objective	Contain, preserve evidence, detain witnesses		Evacuate, decon, preserve evidence, contain		Protect responders, extricate, treat and transport		Conduct intelligence gathering, contain, quarantine	
Secondary Objectives								
Logistics	Red Cross – Food, Water Shelter – Emergency management		Red Cross – Food, water, blankets, shelter		Red Cross – Food, water Medical supplies – EMS		CDC – Vaccines Hospitals – Medical supplies	
Finance	City accountant		City accountant		Budget office		State financial officer Regional financial officers	
Planning	State police or local LEO		Fire department or HazMat rep		Technical rescue team rep		Public health	
Operations	SP or LEO		FD or Hazmat		FD or Tech rescue		Public health or EMS	
Mutual Aid Thresholds	5 fatalities or 25 injured – contact SP		2nd alarm		>3 people trapped, respond second team		> 1,000 cases, request State assistance	
Emergency Declarations	LE decisions		Working incident		Working incident		PH decision	
Disaster Declarations	>25 killed or injured		3rd alarm insufficient		>3 rescue teams required to manage the incident		>10,000 cases, hospitals >105% capacity	
Disaster Declaration Responsibility	Mayor or town administrator		Mayor or town administrator		Mayor or town administrator		Mayor or town administrator	
Contact Information								

Note that the table above is a guideline only; it should not be seen as a barrier to alternative decisions made by onscene command.

Threat Decisions

Generally, planners should focus on events that are the most likely, and those that have the potential to have the largest impact. Planning for events such as structural collapse or hazardous materials releases should only be done if technical teams are involved in the planning and share responsibility for responding to the incident (single all-hazard fire department or multiagency agreement for other EMS delivery models).

EMS mass gathering planners should create plans for threats over which EMS has authority. For instance, if planning the medical aspects of a small concert, and a large fight breaks out, law enforcement will be in charge of the incident. EMS planners should integrate the medical response into the overall law enforcement response strategy.

Review a few of the most likely scenarios and tabletop exercise each scenario using the resources and resource placements chosen. Ask questions such as:

- Do onscene units have sufficient equipment and training to organize for this hazard?
- How many, what type of patients can be treated with resources on site?
- What offsite resources will need to be called in to handle this hazard?
- How do resource requests occur, whose approval is needed, and who will reimburse those resources for their expenses?
- Will emergency operations impede evacuation if needed?
- How might high winds, temperature extremes, or rain affect the area?
- How will communication with responding units occur?
- Where will media personnel be directed? Concerned/Separated family members?

Schedule personnel needed and remember to allow sufficient time for mobilization, briefing, demobilization, and debriefing (or "hotwash"). Have a backup plan if any key personnel become sick or unable to fulfill their roles.

Action Plans

Once risk assessments are complete, planning can begin. Be sure to use existing MCI plans, National Incident Management System (NIMS) guidance, and information in the Emergency Support Function (ESF) annexes to the National Response Plan (NRP) as a starting point for event-specific MCI plans. Excessive variation from the agency's MCI plan and prevailing planning principles will create confusion and training issues.

Experience has demonstrated that plans will likely **not** be adhered to during an actual emergency unless significant time and effort is spent on training personnel. Training on and exercising the plan requires significant investment of time and resources and should be planned for while budgeting and developing personnel management schemes.

To the greatest extent possible, operations plans should not deviate from normal operational procedures. In an emergency, responders are more likely to rely on past training and skills than the guidance in the action plan if the processes and procedures used in the plan vary significantly from normal operations. Lessons learned from the conflicts in Iraq and Afghanistan demonstrate the importance of aligning standard operating procedures with emergency action plans.

Role of Communications Center

- Call takers should carefully prioritize calls.

- Call takers should be familiar with venue landmarks that can be used by callers to identify their location.

- Call takers should identify patients that are ambulatory or have friends or family able to relocate the patient.

- Event personnel should be directed to relocate patients to aid stations or prearranged meeting locations whenever possible. Provide wheelchairs for this purpose whenever practical.

- Develop tools and techniques such as flags or strobe lights to help medical personnel find event personnel that are with a patient.

- Clearly mark aid stations and staging locations.

- EMS personnel should be trained and equipped to care for several patients at once, without other medical assistance.

- Avoid requesting transport when unnecessary. Victims of exhaustion should be provided with shelter, hydration, and provided the opportunity to recover unless life-threatening signs and symptoms are present.

- Have a plan for how mutual aid resources will be used if they are requested.

Relationship of Event Command to Responding Resources

When an MCI occurs at a mass gathering incident, additional local EMS, law enforcement, and fire suppression resources will be dispatched to the event. Unless carefully coordinated, these responding resources are going to establish their own onscene command structure. Planning for a mass gathering must include coordination of command contingencies in the event of an MCI at the event that are consistent with NIMS principles. A Unified Command (UC) can help coordinate the actions of the various departments involved and improve responder safety.

Resource Requests

It is important that onscene command personnel have access to event organizers and those with authority to make decisions on behalf of event personnel. When resources are needed during an MCI, event personnel should be notified when and where these resources will be arriving.

Involving event personnel in resource requests can prevent duplication of services and should make mobilization of event personnel resources more efficient. If event decisionmakers are not present in a command or operations area during the event, redundant communication with those individuals must be available.

Use of Mutual Aid

Mutual aid resources should be used in accordance with existing mutual aid plans. If an event results in the need for additional resources that exceeds the scope of existing mutual aid agreements, planners should engage additional mutual aid partners for the duration of the mass gathering. When assigning tasks or transports to mutual aid resources, attempt to assign them transports that will return them back to their area of operations.

Communications

Significant planning resources must be dedicated to creating communication plans that are sophisticated enough to serve their purpose but simple enough to be usable and reliable. Planners should avoid using any communication system that has not been tested in situ by actual event personnel.

Planners must consider the impact of environmental conditions such as background noise from crowds, loud music, and interference from equipment on radio equipment. Providing the capability for personnel to transmit information accurately under noisy conditions is more challenging than equipping them to receive information in noisy conditions. Special noise cancelling microphones, bone microphones, or laryngophones ("throat mics") may be needed to ensure rescuers are able to transmit in high-noise environments. Planners should consider the use of text paging or text messaging for low-priority communications such as informational updates.

It is important to remember that as the number of radios with access to a channel or talk group increases, the potential for that communication method to be rendered unusable increases as well. Even with trunked radio systems, excessive radio traffic can disable other communications by monopolizing the bandwidth available. One or more channels not accessible or used by most responders should be reserved for critical communications between command personnel (i.e., a command net).

Text messaging, instant messaging, and direct connect technologies all use less cellular bandwidth than conventional voice calls. This may be helpful when cellular networks are overloaded. EMS planners should also determine if cellular priority services such as Government Emergency Telecommunications Service (GETS) are available and/or necessary.

Consider the use of satellite phones if communication with offsite communication centers or individuals is critical. Satellite phones will often provide voice, data, and text messaging capability when local cellular or other networks are disabled. It is also important to consider spare batteries, chargers, and headsets in the planning phase.

Amateur Radio

During emergency situations, most areas of the country have access to Amateur Radio Emergency Services (ARES). These amateur radio enthusiasts volunteer their time, equipment, and expertise to establish emergency communications if more conventional systems are not available. Such groups may also be willing to assist during special events to help provide radio coverage over large event courses with poor conventional radio coverage. Skill levels and sophistication of equipment varies widely and must be assessed before determining whether this would be a good option.

Amateur radio operators may be able to provide voice, facsimile, and various forms of data communications. ARES groups are often able to erect their own antenna towers and provide their own electrical power in remote areas.

Expanded Scope/Emerging Mass Casualty Incident Management Considerations

In the future, Advanced Practice Paramedics may be used on the scene of an MCI to provide a more thorough assessment of ill or injured patients. This more thorough assessment could include abdominal ultrasounds and blood analysis to detect hidden hemorrhages. Such measures could be used to improve triage accuracy during MCIs and provide reassurance to patients and responders that transport is unnecessary for a particular patient. Such skills are normally the domain of doctors of medicine (MDs)/doctors of osteopathy (DOs) and physicians assistants (PAs)/nurse-practitioners (NPs), and these providers would certainly be helpful during MCIs if rapidly available and properly prepared to operate in the field.

Treat and Release protocols could be used to care for minor injuries on scene reducing hospital transports. EMS professionals could provide wound care, breathing treatments, splinting, and printed instructions on when to seek further medical assistance.

Alternative transport destinations are another emerging option for minor injuries and illnesses when local hospitals are being overwhelmed by more serious cases. Spreading transports out to physician offices and urgent care centers is an option that emergency planners should explore in cooperation with emergency management and local medical direction.

Current EMS training and protocols encourage responders to provide care and transport for every individual they encounter who exhibits a chief complaint or has a mechanism of injury. Examination of mass care incidents reveals that resources are expended caring for "patients" who not only have no life threatening injuries, but also often have no injuries at all. This practice inflates patient loads and results in the relocation of the disaster from the field environment to the hospital. Creating a clinically responsible system to discourage the transport of citizens who are not injured or have clearly superficial injuries will limit the impact of the MCI on hospitals and the EMS system as a whole.

Recognizing an MCI Situation

A well-established problem organizing and managing an MCI is recognition that one is occurring. For instance, if a large number of people have been sitting in the sun at an athletic event and are on the verge of heat exhaustion, responders will first respond with two or three calls for "diabetic" or "person fainted." Not until two teams are dispatched to different areas, and several more calls come in, does it become apparent that a tightly packed crowd of people has turned into an MCI situation. The risk is that several teams will be working individual calls without realizing that there is a larger problem.

Differentiating between a surge in patient volume and an actual MCI can be very challenging. Providing operations personnel with preselected thresholds or trigger points for making these determinations can be very helpful. These thresholds may be defined as a particular patient count in a specific period or as the occurrence of a specific event such as activation of mutual aid resources. It is critical that event organizers are involved in these discussions and agree to cancel the event when specific thresholds are met.

Special Considerations
Active Shooter Situations

Active shooter situations are unique and complicated situations that should be planned for in careful coordination with law enforcement entities within the event jurisdiction.

License Reciprocity Issues

License reciprocity issues should be considered based on local and State requirements and discussed with competent medical-legal advisors, EMS regulatory agencies within the jurisdiction, and the State EMS Office within the provider's State.

EMS Equipment on MCI Scenes

EMS supervisors and managers spend a great deal of time and effort ensuring that their crews bring the required equipment into each call they are dispatched on. Providers are often told they must bring their stretcher, jump kit, oxygen, and electrocardiogram (ECG) monitor onto every call to ensure they have the right equipment if a patient's condition turns out to be different from that reported by the 9-1-1 caller. This training may be problematic during an MCI situation.

Ambulance stretchers, especially, should not be removed from an ambulance unless necessary. Ambulance stretchers require two trained operators and are difficult to maneuver in buildings and across uneven ground. In addition, significant delays can be caused when attempting to load patients into an ambulance with a missing stretcher or a stretcher that doesn't fit in the stretcher mounts. A better alternative is to use pole stretchers, wheelchairs, or back boards to move nonambulatory patients.

Freelancing

Freelancing should not be tolerated during training or during actual incidents. Freelancing leads to confusion, poor personnel accountability, and often leads to providers being injured because they are not equipped or briefed for the hazards present on scene. Freelancers that arrive in vehicles also have effectively placed a roadblock wherever they parked their vehicle. If a vehicle is left in a location which blocks emergency vehicle ingress or egress, law enforcement should be prepared to have the vehicle towed as quickly as possible. Security/Law enforcement personnel staffing the perimeter of an incident should be instructed to direct any personnel attempting to enter the scene to the staging area. Law enforcement personnel should be briefed on contingencies to deal with personnel who refuse to operate within established parameters and interfere with emergency operations.

Traffic Flow

It is important that law enforcement, department of transportation, and/or public works agencies be enlisted early during an incident to ensure that responding emergency vehicles have both ingress and egress routes available to them, while all unnecessary vehicles and traffic be routed away from the area. If a vehicle is left in a location which blocks emergency vehicle ingress or egress, law enforcement should be prepared to have the vehicle towed as quickly as possible.

Mass Casualty Incident Planning Checklist

- ❏ Gather all available historical records on the event
    - ❏ Computer-aided dispatch (CAD) data
    - ❏ Attendance data
    - ❏ Previous Operations (OPS) plans
    - ❏ Previous After Action Reports (AARs)
- ❏ List the stakeholders and make contact with them
- ❏ Meet with event organizers, schedule periodic updates
- ❏ Define and map the event area of operations
    - ❏ Locate evacuation points
    - ❏ Locate emergency ingress and egress points
    - ❏ Locate potential aid station locations
    - ❏ Locate potential equipment caches
    - ❏ Identify highly visible landmarks that can be used by callers to identify their location
    - ❏ Identify potential areas for establishment of treatment and transportation areas
- ❏ Document all ambulance providers' (air and land) contact information and capabilities in area around event
- ❏ Perform risk assessment
- ❏ Determine level of security to use in planning and operations
- ❏ Create threat-specific plans
    - ❏ Possible command structure
    - ❏ Likely resource requests
    - ❏ Determination as to whether incident will be commanded by onscene event staff or responding resources
    - ❏ Create a generic plan for threats not addressed or anticipated
- ❏ Create contact information cards
    - ❏ For command personnel
    - ❏ For security
    - ❏ For EMS personnel
    - ❏ For other event staff

- Perform a walk-through of the event location with event organizers. Update map locations as necessary
- Test radio communication equipment at the event location
    - Search for and document areas of poor reception
    - Test every channel that will be used during event
    - Verify interoperability of agency radios if this is important to your communication plan
    - Test cell phone reception using provider-specific phones
- Determine best location for event operations post, if applicable, based on following criteria
    - Cell phone reception
    - Access to landline telephones
    - Broadband internet access—test with computers to be used during actual event
    - Radio reception
    - Access to toilet facilities
    - Isolation from high-noise environments

Incident Action Plan Safety and Risk Analysis, ICS Form 215A

INCIDENT ACTION PLAN SAFETY ANALYSIS	1. Incident Name							2. Date	3. Time
Division or Group	**Potential Hazards**							**Mitigations** (e.g., PPE, buddy system, escape routes)	
	Type of Hazard:	Type of Hazard:	Type of Hazard:	Type of Hazard:	Type of Hazard:	Type of Hazard:	Type of Hazard:		
Prepared by (Name and Position)									

This page was intentionally left blank.

SECTION V: Policy Guidance for Emergency Medical Services Aspects of Mass Shelter and Feeding

Emergency Medical Services Participation in Mass Shelter and Feeding

Pearlington, MS, is a Census Designated Place with a base population of 1,600 residents located on the border between Mississippi and Louisiana. On August 29, 2005, at 10 a.m. Central Daylight Time (CDT), Hurricane Katrina made landfall at Pearlington. The storm surge, which measured between 12 and 20 feet, continued 4.5 miles inland. With the exception of two homes, every building in the community sustained severe structural damage or was completely destroyed. With its infrastructure destroyed, the local volunteer Fire Chief established a food and water distribution point and a hasty outdoor camp to serve as a shelter. During the first 5 days of the event, the facilities established by the Fire Chief were the primary sources of food, water, and shelter in Pearlington. A four soldier element of the Florida National Guard, an engine company with four firefighters from Bradenton, FL, and an ambulance from Troy, MI, with two Paramedics arrived to conduct search and rescue and provide support on September 1. On September 2, a shelter was established at the elementary school that served a transient population of near 600 people. Follow on support for the community continued to arrive over the next 10 days.

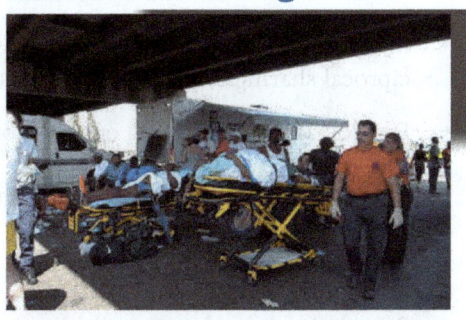

Evacuees with health or medical problems are examined in a triage area set up at a main staging site.

Emergency Medical Services (EMS) agencies fill an important role in ensuring a safe and healthy environment for evacuees living in shelters as a result of a mass incident. A sampling of roles that EMS agencies have fulfilled in mass shelter and feeding operations include:

- Identifying shelter sites in the community in cooperation with public health authorities.

- Providing onsite medical care and first aid at the shelter.

- Supplementing Federal Disaster Medical Assistance Team (DMAT) or Medical Reserve Corps (MRC) assets at an identified shelter.

- Managing shelter operations in cooperation with the American Red Cross (ARC), local emergency management, or local public health authorities.

- Responding to shelters to manage onsite medical emergencies that exceed the capabilities of shelter medical staff.

National Response Framework

Mass care shelters are addressed in Emergency Support Function 6 (ESF-6)–Mass Care, Emergency Assistance, Housing, and Human Services of the National Response Framework and in similar ESF guidance within State emergency management plans.

Summary of Shelter Operations for Emergency Medical Services

Mass shelter operations are ideally organized under the same incident management principles found in the National Incident Management System (NIMS). Using a scalable system, shelters will have need for planning and leadership within the functional roles of Administration, Finance, Logistics, and Operations at a minimum. EMS leaders must understand how the classic Incident Command System (ICS) roles are adapted within the mass shelter environment, particularly Administration, Logistics, and Operations.

Key Functional Roles and Tasks

Administration

- The Administration function at the shelter is responsible to:

- Monitor local media including radio, television, and official sources.

- Maintain close and ongoing contact with the local Emergency Operations Center (EOC) to ensure a reciprocal sharing of planning information.

- Develop action plans based on the information above and from information gathered at planning meetings.

- Work with the shelter manager in planning for anticipated shelter needs and in planning for the next 24 to 48 hours of shelter activity.

- Plan staffing schedules and determining staffing rotations.

- Provide information on available recovery assistance (especially information on the availability of temporary or long-term housing); keep information up-to-date and post in a visible place for shelter residents (e.g., bulletin boards).

- Keep a disaster activity log with detailed records of meetings, decisions, and actions (e.g., who made what decisions).

- Record important interagency contacts and agreements. This is vital for after action reports and for future planning.

- Support information needs related to helping reunite family members.

- Assist nonprofit and governmental agencies with the recruitment, placement, and management of spontaneous disaster volunteers.

- Identify Volunteer Organizations Active in Disasters (VOAD) agencies.

- Translate documents into other languages or to find bilingual individuals to communicate with non-English speaking persons.
    - Find trained Sign Language Interpreters to communicate with deaf persons.

- Coordinate demobilization activities at the conclusion of the deployment.

Logistics

The Logistics function at the shelter works in close coordination with the Logistics Section at the local EOC to accomplish the following:

- Obtain all resources necessary to operate the shelter facility in coordination with the EOC Logistics Section.
    - personnel;
    - food;
    - transportation;
    - supplies and equipment;

- communication resources; and
- all other personal services as applicable for shelter residents (health, mental health, translation, etc.).

• Work with the Finance Coordinator to set up vendor agreements with local businesses as necessary for the purchase of supplies and equipment to operate the shelter.

Operations

The operations function in a mass shelter should work within the definitions provided for the Operations role under NIMS. In addition, specific roles needed to operate a mass care shelter are described below.

Registration: The Registration function ensures that basic data identifying each shelter occupant is collected upon admission to the shelter. A key function of this element is identification of shelter occupants that may have special medical or dietary needs in addition to identifying any potential occupant that may pose a security concern.

Dining Facility (DFAC): The Dining Facility function is responsible for planning, preparing, and distributing all meals provided to evacuees. EMS agencies are unlikely to fulfill this role but should be familiar with the general principles and tasks associated with the role.

Bivouac/Barracks: The Bivouac/Barracks function is responsible for layout and management of the portion of the shelter used for sleeping. This includes allocating adequate space for each resident. The formula used by the ARC is to attempt to provide 40 square feet per person for the purpose of sleep quarters and necessary personal items. Bivouac personnel must also remain alert for signs of illness among residents, suspicious behavior, or hazards that may pose risk to the safety of shelter residents.

Health and Medical Services: This is the most likely role for EMS personnel in a mass shelter environment. The Health and Medical Services function provides both primary first aid and emergency care as well as disease prevention and surveillance within the shelter. This includes overseeing the medical needs of any special needs residents and ensuring access to other health care services as needed.

Safety/Security Services: The Safety and Security Services function is responsible for safeguarding the staff, ensuring orderly behavior among shelter residents, crime prevention, and crowd control among others. This function is unlikely to be delegated to EMS personnel and is most commonly executed by law enforcement or via contract with private security companies.

Transportation Services: The Transportation function is responsible for assisting residents of the area impacted by the incident with basic transport needs including help with transportation to the shelter, transportation from the shelter to access services, and emergency transportation if needed. The transportation function will also assist with distribution of food and supplies in the community in coordination with the EOC.

OPERATIONS BASIC TASK CHECKLIST: MASS SHELTER

GENERAL TASKS

COMPLETE	ELEMENT
	Inspect the facility for safety hazards.
	Restrict access to unsafe areas and any area that will not be in use.
	Establish communication with EOC in the jurisdiction if not already in place.
	Report shelter status, personnel, and equipment needs to Command.
	Designate a staging area if not already in place.
	Assign available staff to shelter operational roles.
	Prepare or assign the preparation of briefings for each operational period.
	Prepare or assign the preparation of relevant ICS Forms.
	Monitor news outlets and official sources for information relating to the incident.

REGISTRATION TASKS

COMPLETE	ELEMENT
	Define a space for registration.
	Set up a registration table and chairs.
	Post a sign directing evacuees to the registration area.
	Post a sign prohibiting possession of weapons, alcohol, or illegal drugs at the shelter.
	Post a sign prohibiting pets at the shelter if applicable.
	Ensure adequate supply of registration forms.
	Establish a log for residents to sign in and out of the shelter.

DINING FACILITY TASKS

COMPLETE	ELEMENT
	Inspect the food preparation area at the shelter site.
	Obtain access to food storage areas.
	Determine if cooking equipment is still functioning and is safe to use.
	Coordinate with Logistics or identified source to ensure food supplies.
	Define a system for managing food waste.
	Define a system for managing food spoilage.
	Define a system for ensuring sanitary food preparation guidelines are followed.
	Establish a system for instituting multiple seating times if warranted by shelter size.
	Identify any resident that has any special dietary needs (diabetic, gluten free diet, etc.).
	Establish a dining area.
	Post a sign designating meal times.
	Recruit residents to prepare food if needed.
	Establish a log of meals served.
	Log all supplies and food ordered and used with applicable receipts.

Section V: Policy Guidance for Emergency Medical Service Aspects of Mass Shelter and Feeding

OPERATIONS BASIC TASK CHECKLIST: MASS SHELTER

BIVOUAC/BARRACKS TASKS

COMPLETE	ELEMENT
	Inspect the Bivouac/Barracks area for hazards to shelter residents.
	Coordinate with Logistics or identified source to ensure adequate sleeping/personal supplies.
	Set up sleeping areas.
	Distribute blankets, mats, and personal items as needed.
	Ensure adequate ventilation.
	Recruit residents to assist with routine cleaning and maintaining an orderly environment.
	Post quiet/lights out hours and any other rules for the facility.
	Monitor the Bivouac area for safety/security issues.

HEALTH AND MEDICAL SERVICES

COMPLETE	ELEMENT
	Inspect the Health and Medical Services area for hazards to shelter residents.
	Coordinate with Logistics or identified source to ensure adequate medical supplies.
	Set up seats and cots to facilitate patient treatment.
	Ensure 24 hour availability of staff (schedule, onsite call, etc.).
	Define a system for recall of off duty on site personnel in the event of patient surge.
	Define how medical emergencies that require offsite care will be handled.
	Document all care according to local rules and procedure.
	Define a system for notifying public health officials if a disease outbreak is identified.
	Identify an area that could serve as an isolation ward should the need arise.

SAFETY/SECURITY SERVICES

COMPLETE	ELEMENT
	Conduct inspection of entire facility at least daily for hazards to shelter residents.
	Ensures shelter is operated according to fire code.
	Maintains clear paths to all exits.
	Ensures fire extinguishers are present and operational.
	Conducts patrol of shelter to reduce opportunity for criminal behavior.
	Coordinates management of any criminal matters with EOC and law enforcement.
	Maintains a log of any suspicious behavior or suspected criminal activity.

TRANSPORTATION SERVICES

COMPLETE	ELEMENT
	Coordinate need for transportation services with emergency Operations Center.
	Determine number and type of transportation resources needed.
	Coordinate the request for resources with the Emergency Operations Center.
	Log the number and type of resources requested on the appropriate ICS form.
	Establish staging area for transportation resources.
	Institute check in and check out procedures to ensure personnel accountability.
	Create a log of all persons transported into or out of the shelter.

Mass Shelter and Feeding Resources

California Emergency Medical Services Authority	http://www.emsa.ca.gov/disaster/default.asp
South Carolina Emergency Management Division	http://www.scemd.org/Prepare/index.html
State of Louisiana Governor's Office of Homeland Security and Emergency Preparedness	http://gohsep.la.gov/
Florida Division of Emergency Management	http://www.floridadisaster.org/internet_library.htm#response
State of Washington Military Department	http://www.emd.wa.gov/
American Red Cross	http://www.redcross.org/
National Volunteer Organizations Active in Disaster	http://www.nvoad.org/
National Organization on Disability	http://www.nod.org/research_publications/emergency_preparedness_materials/
The Salvation Army	http://disaster.salvationarmyusa.org/

SECTION VI: Local Mutual Aid

TEMPLATE: Local, Regional, and State Mutual Aid

Introduction

Mutual aid agreements and memorandums of understanding (MOU) are written documents describing how personnel, equipment, facilities, and/or supplies will be requested, made available, and used by or between organizations, agencies, or jurisdictions. These agreements are necessary due to the likelihood that system volume from multiple responses or a single large scale emergency response will exceed the ability of endogenous assets to meet the needs of the system. Examples of incidents that can cause system overload include multiple-alarm fires, traffic accidents with injuries, and criminal acts including terrorism.

Mutual aid may also extend beyond local response. Several States have statewide mutual aid systems, examples include Washington and Oregon statewide mobilization programs. Mutual Aid Box Alarm System (MABAS) is a regional mutual aid system, headquartered in Illinois, with 1,500 member fire departments in Illinois, Indiana, Wisconsin, Iowa, and Missouri. (See Annex V.)

Mutual aid may be planned so that it is triggered by a requesting agency at the time the system is overloaded. Mutual aid may also take the form of a standing agreement for cooperative emergency management on a continuing basis. In that model, resource deployment is planned based on conditional variables, such as ensuring that resources are dispatched from the nearest fire station, regardless of which side of a jurisdictional boundary the incident is on. Agreements that send the closest resources are regularly referred to as automatic aid agreements. Automatic aid agreements and mutual aid agreements are established through legal covenants between jurisdictions.

The key difference between a mutual aid agreement and an MOU is that mutual aid agreements pledge reciprocal assistance of a particular type and definition between two or more organizations, agencies, or jurisdictions. An MOU can be reciprocal in nature, with parties agreeing to help one another under certain terms, or an MOU can pledge assistance to an organization, agency, or jurisdiction without mutual benefit.

A plan to use external organizations, agencies, or jurisdictions is a routine part of Emergency Medical Services (EMS) system planning and forms the basis of surge response strategy. To ensure that there is clear understanding by all parties agreeing to provide mutual aid or external assistance in cooperation with outside agencies, a written mutual aid agreement or MOU should be executed by authorized representatives from both the agency providing and the agency receiving the resources.

The following elements or provisions should be included in mutual aid agreements and MOUs.

COMPLETE	Local and Regional Mutual Aid Checklist
	ELEMENT
	Consistent with NIMS and State level Incident Management Systems.
	Describes agency location.
	Definitions of key terms used in the agreement.
	Roles and responsibilities of individual parties.
	Requires minimum levels of training based on roles.
	Provides for recognition of qualifications and certifications.
	Describes procedures for requesting and providing assistance.
	Describes a system for mobilization and deployment of resources.
	Describes resources available for daily mutual aid response by day and time.
	Describes resources available for Mass Incident response by day and time.
	Describes resources other than EMS agencies (Red Cross, bus system, etc.).
	Define a system for determining which resources will be used in which order.
	Describes jurisdictional specifics (demographics, resources, risks, etc.).
	Describe seasonal and temporal factors that impact the agreement.
	Addresses coverage of the assisting agency area while providing mutual aid.
	Addresses communication between agencies while providing mutual aid.
	Addresses personnel safety.
	Addresses liability protection.
	Addresses reimbursement for services.
	Addresses protocol and clinical oversight if applicable.
	Addresses post incident critical stress management.
	Addresses the use of After Action Review to improve the plan.
	Requires review of the plan annually or more often as needed.
	Defines a method for updating the plan to maintain operational relevance.
	Describes a method for communicating changes in the agreement.

TEMPLATE: Inter-Local Government Agreement–Mutual Aid

<INSERT JURISDICTION HERE> Mutual Aid

Inter-Local Government Agreement ("Agreement")

Recitals

WHEREAS

The counties, cities, towns, townships, fire protection **<INSERT JURISDICTION HERE>** and other relevant entities (collectively referred to as "Signatories to this Agreement" or "Signatories") of **<INSERT JURISDICTION HERE>** desire to enter into this Agreement for the purposes of providing for mutual support, aid, and assistance between the signatories following the occurrence of a natural or manmade disaster emergency and for conducting preparation activities including but not limited to planning, training, exercises, response, grant applications, and other resource coordination.

Articles

NOW, THEREFORE, the parties hereby agree as follows:

Article I: Definitions

Assisting Jurisdiction: A jurisdiction participating in the Agreement and providing emergency response manpower, equipment, and resources to another jurisdiction that has requested assistance to confront an emergency.

Authorized Representative: The chief executive of a participating jurisdiction, or his or her designee, who has authorization to request, offer, or provide assistance under the terms of this Agreement.

Emergency Management Agency (EMA): The agency which manages emergency preparedness and response on a countywide basis.

Director Emergency Management (DEM): The position that manages the emergency management agency or his or her designee.

Emergency: Any occurrence, or threat thereof, whether natural or caused by man, in war or in peace, which results or may result in substantial injury or harm to the population, substantial damage to or loss of property, or substantial harm to the environment and is beyond the capacity of an individual jurisdiction to effectively control.

Mutual Aid: A prearranged written agreement and plan whereby assistance is requested and provided between two or more jurisdictions during a designated emergency under terms of the Agreement.

Period of Assistance: The period of time beginning with the departure of any personnel and/or equipment of the assisting jurisdiction from any point for the purpose of traveling to provide assistance exclusively to the requesting jurisdiction, and ending on the return of all of the assisting jurisdiction's personnel and equipment to their regular place of work or assignment, or otherwise terminated through written or verbal notice to the authorized representative of the requesting jurisdiction by the authorized representative of the assisting jurisdiction.

Requesting Jurisdiction: A jurisdiction under an emergency condition that has requested assistance from another jurisdiction participating in the Agreement.

Staging Area: A location identified outside the immediate emergency area where emergency response equipment and personnel assemble for briefing, assignment, and related matters.

Article II: Terms of the Agreement

Activation

1. The Signatories of **<INSERT JURISDICTION HERE>** [ ] agree that any assistance which may be furnished under this Agreement from one party to the other shall not be regarded as "available assets" of the requesting party for purposes of determining whether local assets are sufficient or insufficient to respond to any natural or manmade emergency or disaster.

2. Each party agrees that in the event of an emergency situation, each other party to this Agreement will furnish such personnel, equipment, facilities or services as are available, provided that such action would not unreasonably diminish the capacity to provide basic services to its own jurisdiction.

3. The Signatories of **<INSERT JURISDICTION HERE>** [ ] agree that the senior officers (and their assistants, or alternatives) of the entities that will provide direct assistance under this Agreement (i.e., fire chief, sheriff, police chief, EMS provider, highway superintendent, Emergency Support Function (ESF) Coordinator, etc.) shall be accorded the status of emergency management personnel for purposes of administration of this Agreement. The senior officers in command of the units providing assistance under this Agreement are required to promptly inform the DEM and the appropriate chief executive of their respective unit of government that the assets have been sent out of the area. This step will allow the DEM to keep track of assets remaining for response to other emergencies that might arise while mutual aid assistance is being rendered.

4. The chief executive or his or her designee of each participating jurisdiction to this Agreement shall act as the authorized representative of that jurisdiction. If the chief executive or his or her designee is not available, the official next in the line of succession as defined by local or State statute shall assume responsibilities of the authorized representative. The name, title, jurisdiction, county, and contact information for each of the authorized representatives is attached to this Agreement and labeled Authorized Representatives.

5. The Signatories of **<INSERT JURISDICTION HERE>** [ ] agree that their respective county EMAs shall be the entities which are appropriate to administer and call into effect the activation terms of this Agreement pursuant to the subsequent provisions.

6. To invoke assistance under the provisions of this Agreement, the authorized representative from the Requesting Jurisdiction shall be required to contact the DEM or his or her designee of the county in which the requesting jurisdiction resides. This communication may be conducted by telephone, in writing, or via email or other electronic communication.

7. Each request for assistance shall be accompanied by the following information, to the extent known:

    - A general description of the damage or injury sustained or threatened;

    - Identification of the emergency service function or functions for which assistance is needed (e.g., fire, law enforcement, emergency medical, search and rescue, transportation, communications, public works and engineering, building, inspection, planning and information assistance, mass care, resource support, health and other medical services, etc.) and the particular type of assistance needed;

- The amount and type of personnel, equipment, materials, supplies, and/or facilities needed and a reasonable estimate of the period of assistance that each will be needed;

- The location or locations to which the resources are to be dispatched and the specific time by which the resources are needed; and

- The name and contact information of a representative of the Requesting Party to meet the personnel and equipment of any Assisting Party at each location to which resources are dispatched.

This information may be provided on a form designed for this purpose or by any other available means.

8. The DEM shall forward the request for assistance to DEMs in the appropriate counties within the **<INSERT JURISDICTION HERE>** based on the proximity and availability of the resources required by the request. The DEMs who receive a request for assistance shall contact the Authorized Representatives of the local jurisdictions within the county and submit the request for assistance.

9. A DEM who determines that his or her Assisting Jurisdictions have the available personnel, equipment, or other resources, shall so notify the DEM of the Requesting Jurisdiction and provide the following information, to the extent known:

- A complete description of the personnel and their expertise and capabilities, equipment, and other resources to be furnished to the Requesting Party;

- The estimated period of assistance that the personnel, equipment, and other resources will be available;

- The name of the person or persons to be designated as supervisory personnel for the Assisting Jurisdiction; and

- The estimated time of arrival for the assistance to be provided at the designated location.

This information may be provided on a form designed for this purpose or by any other available means.

Incident Command

10. The parties shall use the Incident Command System (ICS) as developed by the U.S. Department of Homeland Security (DHS) as part of the National Incident Management System (NIMS) to provide structure for incident management so as to assure efficient use of resources and the safety of emergency responders and the public.

11. During an emergency situation, all personnel from the Assisting Jurisdictions shall report to and work under the direction of the designated Incident Commander (IC). Personnel from either the Requesting or Assisting Jurisdiction may receive supervision from any command personnel from the combined participating jurisdictions if authorized by the IC or her or his designee in the command structure. Tactical teams shall operate under the direction of their tactical commander once they are authorized to undertake assignments.

Liability

12. Pursuant to **<INSERT STATE CODE HERE>** the chief executive of the political subdivision which is the Assisting Jurisdiction in this agreement may assign or make available for duty the appropriate emergency response personnel outside of the physical limits of their political subdivision; and pursuant to **<INSERT STATE CODE HERE>**, when Homeland Security, Emergency Management, or Emergency Support

Functions are so ordered to render aid outside the physical limits of their political subdivision, they will retain the same powers, duties, rights, privileges and immunities including any coverage under the Worker's Compensation Laws, that they receive when they are on duty in their home jurisdiction.

13. The party who requests mutual aid shall in no way be deemed liable or responsible for the personal property of the members of the responding party which may be lost, stolen, or damaged while performing their duties in responding under the terms of this Agreement.

14. The Assisting Jurisdictions under the terms of this Agreement shall assume no responsibility or liability for property damaged or destroyed or bodily injury at the actual scene of any emergency due to actions which are required in responding under this Agreement; said liability and responsibility shall rest solely with the jurisdiction requesting such aid and within whose boundaries the property exists or the incident occurs.

15. Pursuant to **<INSERT STATE CODE HERE>** the political subdivision that constitutes the Requesting Jurisdiction shall be responsible for any loss or damage to equipment used in the response and shall pay any expense incurred in the operation and maintenance thereof as well as any expense incurred in the provision of a service or other expenses in answering the request for assistance.

16. Each of the parties agree that each Assisting Jurisdiction shall provide for the payment of compensation and benefits to:

    - an injured member; and

    - a representative of a deceased member

    of the Assisting Jurisdiction's emergency forces if the member is injured or killed while rendering assistance under this Agreement in the same manner and on the same terms as if the injury or death were sustained while the member was rendering assistance for or within the member's own jurisdiction. Expenses incurred for such compensation or benefits shall not be reimbursable pursuant to other provisions in this Agreement.

17. Should there be any disagreement as to the nature and extent of any provision pertaining to liability, these issues shall be submitted to binding arbitration with the American Arbitration Association or any other arbitration association unanimously agreed to by the parties involved in the dispute.

18. The execution of this Agreement shall not give rise to any liability or responsibility for failure to respond to any request for assistance made pursuant to this Agreement. This Agreement shall not be construed as or deemed to be an Agreement for the benefit of any third party or parties, and no third party or parties shall have any right of action whatsoever hereunder for any cause whatsoever.

Conditions of Participation

19. Interagency and interjurisdictional plans shall be developed as necessary and in compliance with State and Federal mandates; they shall be updated on a regular basis by the parties hereto and are operative among the parties in accordance with such plans.

20. The parties agree to meet on a regular basis to review all assistance plans and the provisions of this Agreement.

21. This Agreement shall become effective when approved and executed by the lawful representative of each participating party. This Agreement shall remain in effect as between and among each and every

party until participation in this Agreement is terminated by a party in writing. Termination of participation in this Agreement by a party shall not affect the continued operation of this Agreement between and among the remaining parties. Any party to this Agreement may terminate participation in this Agreement upon thirty (30) days' written notice addressed to the fiscal agent for **<INSERT JURISDICTION HERE>** [ ].

Reimbursement

22. An itemized claim for loss and damage to the responding party's equipment at the response scene shall be filed within thirty (30) days of such loss or damage occurring. (NOTE: Filing within thirty days will help to ensure Federal Emergency Management Agency (FEMA) reimbursement, if applicable.)

23. The political subdivision in which the requested party is located shall be responsible for labor and equipment reimbursement as specified in item 25 in this Agreement.

24. The parties agree that, as specified in **<INSERT STATE CODE HERE>**, no claim for loss, damage, or expense under this Agreement shall be allowed unless, within thirty (30) days after the same is sustained or incurred, an itemized notice of such claim under oath is served by mail or otherwise upon the Chief Fiscal Officer of such political subdivision where the equipment was used. Claims shall be fully documented in order to obtain reimbursement for State and Federal DHS reimbursement funds when and if available.

25. The parties agree that labor and equipment reimbursement rates shall be as follows:

- Labor rates:
  - Straight time for force account labor shall be the normal pay rates for responding personnel.
  - Overtime for force account labor shall be at 1 1/2 times the normal pay rates for responding personnel if it is the normal practice to pay overtime at this rate.
  - Volunteer Note: Under FEMA 9523.6 Section 7.B.3. "If the providing (Assisting Jurisdiction) entity is staffed with volunteer labor, the value of the volunteer labor may be credited to the non-Federal cost share in accordance with the provisions of the Donated Resources policy (#9525.2).
- Equipment reimbursement rates:
  - Equipment reimbursement rates shall be at the FEMA standard for equipment reimbursement or the State or local rate, whichever is lowest.

IN WITNESS WHEREOF, this Agreement has been executed and approved and is effective and operative as to each of the parties as herein provided as of the day and year written below.

[DATED, NAME, TITLE AND SIGNATURE OF EACH PARTICIPATING JURISDICTION]

Additional Sample Agreements

Additional sample mutual aid agreements are located in Annex I.

This page was intentionally left blank.

ANNEX I: Sample Mutual Aid Agreements

EXAMPLE: Single County Mutual Aid Agreement

Description

This sample mutual aid agreement from the State of Idaho is intended to improve coordination between emergency responders across the public safety spectrum within a single county. Emergency Medical Services (EMS) is addressed directly in the agreement.

**MUTUAL AID AND CONTINGENCY AGREEMENT
BY AND AMONG THE
MEMBERS OF THE XXXXXXXXXX COUNTY EMERGENCY
MEDICAL SERVICES ASSOCIATION**

This agreement is made and entered into effective on the ____ day of _____, 20XX, by and among the Members of the XXXXXXXXXX County Emergency Medical Services Association who have duly executed this Agreement.

WHEREAS, the Members of the XXXXXXXXXX County Emergency Medical Services Association recognize the necessity to cooperate and work together to provide for mutual aid and contingency assistance; and

WHEREAS, the Members further recognize the need to provide for an organized means of resolving conflicts, concerns, and questions between and among their respective Members.

NOW, THEREFORE, IT IS AGREED BY AND AMONG THE MEMBERS WHO HAVE DULY EXECUTED THIS AGREEMENT AS FOLLOWS:

SECTION 1. Definitions:

As used herein:

a. "Requesting Member" shall mean the Member requesting aid, and

b. "Responding Member" shall mean the Member affording or responding to a call for aid.

SECTION 2. Mutual Aid and Contingency Agreement:

The Members of the XXXXXXXXXX County EMS Association mutually agree to provide mutual aid and contingency service to each other.

SECTION 3. Authority to Respond to Provide Assistance:

a. The authority to make requests for assistance or to provide aid under this Agreement shall reside with the requesting Member's command personnel or the command personnel's designee. For purposes of this Agreement, the "requesting Member" shall mean the incident commander or the incident commander's designee asking for assistance and the "responding Member" shall mean an officer/supervisor or designee sending assistance. Any Member shall have the right to request assistance from the other Member's subject to the terms and conditions of this Agreement.

b. The XXXXXXXXXX County Emergency Communications Center will page out the next nearest Member if two consecutive pages go unanswered for any reason. Members are empowered to set up automatic aid protocols in the Emergency Communications Center for specific circumstances in their service areas.

SECTION 4. Requesting Assistance:
A Member may request assistance from any other Member when the requesting Member has concluded that such assistance is essential to protect life.

SECTION 5. Responses to Request:
Upon request, a responding Member, upon determination that an emergency exists and subject to the availability of human and equipment resources, shall dispatch EMS personnel and equipment to aid the requesting Member.

SECTION 6. Personnel and Equipment Provided:
The requesting Member shall include in its request for assistance the amount and type of equipment, and shall specify the location where the personnel and equipment are needed.

The final decision on the amount and type of equipment to be sent shall be solely that of the responding Member. The responding Member shall be immune from any liability in connection with all acts associated herewith provided that the final decision is made with reasonable diligence.

No Member shall make any claim whatsoever against another Member for refusal to send the requested personnel or equipment where such refusal is based on the judgment of the responding Member that such personnel and equipment are either not available or are needed to provide service in the Member's response area.

SECTION 7. Command and Control at the Emergency Scene:
All Members have established Incident Command System (ICS) Standard Operating Procedures (SOPs) and will implement them on all incidents involving mutual aid or contingency responses.

The responding Member's personnel shall report and the equipment shall be given to the incident commander or other appropriate sector officer of the requesting Member. The person in charge of the responding Member shall meet with the incident commander or appropriate sector officer of the requesting Member for a briefing and assignment.

The person in charge of the responding Member shall retain control of the responding Member's human and equipment resources and shall direct them to meet the needs and tasks assigned by the incident commander or sector officer. The responding Member's personnel and equipment shall be released by the requesting Member when the services of the responding Member are no longer required or when the responding Member's resources are needed in their primary response area. Responding Member personnel and equipment may withdraw from the EMS scene upon giving notice to the incident commander or appropriate sector officer that they are needed in the Member's primary response area. It is understood that the purpose of this section is to maintain order at the emergency scene and shall not be construed to establish an employer/employee relationship.

SECTION 8. Reporting and Recordkeeping:

The requesting Member shall maintain records regarding the frequency of the use of this agreement and provide them to the Iowa Department of Public Health Bureau of Emergency Medical Services upon request. Each Member shall maintain individual patient care reports.

SECTION 9. No Reimbursement for Costs:

No Member shall be required to reimburse any other Member for the cost of providing the services set forth in this Agreement for mutual aid services, except as provided in Section 10 below. Each Member shall pay its own costs (i.e., salaries, repairs, materials, compensation, etc.) for responding for requests for mutual aid or contingency response.

SECTION 10. Fees for EMS Agency:

Members providing ambulance transport or other services normally billed for will be entitled to their normal fees for service and are responsible for their own billing, insurance filing and collection activity. Requesting Members are responsible for payment of fees for responding paramedic Members providing paramedic intercept services.

SECTION 11. Liability:

Each responding Member hereby waives all claims against each requesting Member for compensation for any property loss or damage and/or personal injury or death occurring as a consequence of the performance of this Agreement. A responding Member assumes all liability and/or cost of damage to its equipment and the injury or death of its personnel when responding or performing under this agreement.

SECTION 12. Insurance:

Each Member shall procure and maintain such insurance as is required by applicable Federal and State law and as may be appropriate and reasonable to cover its staff, equipment, vehicles, and property, including but not limited to liability insurance, workers' compensation (if applicable), unemployment insurance, automobile liability, and property damage. Members may self-insure when appropriate.

SECTION 13. Conflict Resolution:

From time to time, personnel from one Member or another may have some concerns or questions regarding this Agreement or the working relationship of the parties. Should any such issues arise, they should be dealt with by the Member's chain of command to provide answers or resolution.

SECTION 14. Term of Agreement:

This Agreement shall be in full force and effect upon execution by all Members hereto. This Agreement shall remain in effect for a period of 10 years unless cancelled by any Member by giving 30 days written notice to the XXXXXXXXXX County EMS Association. The Agreement may be amended by agreement of all of the Members.

IN WITNESS THEREOF, the following Members have duly executed this Agreement:

Editor's Note: Signatures deleted

EXAMPLE: Single State Mutual Aid Compact

Description

This sample mutual aid agreement from the State of Alabama is intended to improve coordination between agencies across the healthcare spectrum and the Alabama Department of Public Health. EMS is included as an "Other Healthcare Entity" within this agreement.

MUTUAL AID COMPACT

This Mutual Aid Compact ("Compact") is made and entered into as of this _____ day of _____, 20 _____, by and between ("the Participating Entity") and the Alabama Department of Public Health (ADPH) as compact coordinator. The Compact will remain in effect indefinitely unless terminated by one of the signing parties. The Participating Entity, Other Health Care Entities and Other Entities are collectively referred to as the "Participating Entities."

RECITALS

WHEREAS, this Compact is a statement of principles and procedures which signify the belief and commitment of the Participating Entities that in the event of a disaster as herein below defined, the public health and medical needs of the citizens in Alabama and contiguous States will be best met if the Participating Entities cooperate with one another and coordinate their response efforts; and,

WHEREAS, by signing herein below, all parties understand and acknowledge that no Participating Entity, other health care entity or other entity is bound to provide or accept patients, staff, equipment or supplies; and,

WHEREAS, the terms of this compact apply only in the event and to the extent that such parties utilize and coordinate through AIMS which provides the executing mechanism for the compact; and,

WHEREAS, the Participating Entities desire to set forth the basic tenets of a cooperative and coordinated response plan to facilitate the immediate sharing of regional resources in the event of a disaster; and,

WHEREAS, the Participating Entities acknowledge that any Participating Entity may from time to time find it necessary to evacuate and/or transfer and/or participate in the evacuation or transfer of patients because of the occurrence of a disaster; and,

WHEREAS, the Participating Entities further acknowledge that any Participating Entity may from time to time lack the staff, equipment, supplies and other essential services to optimally meet the needs of patients because of the occurrence of a disaster; and,

WHEREAS, each Participating Entity acknowledges that at any time it may, as a result of a disaster, (i) need assistance as an Affected Entity or (ii) be able to render aid as an Assisting Entity; and,

WHEREAS, the Participating Entities have determined that a Mutual Aid Compact, developed prior to a sudden and immediate disaster, is needed to facilitate communication between the Participating Entities and to coordinate the transfer of patients and the sharing of staff, equipment, supplies and other essential services in the event of a disaster; and,

WHEREAS, Participating Entities recognize that a disaster may impact entities in both Alabama and in contiguous States and may desire to extend the Mutual Aid Compact to include entities in contiguous States that wish to participate in a coordinated response.

NOW THEREFORE, in consideration of the above recitals, the Participating Entities agree as follows:

ARTICLE I

DEFINED TERMS

1.1 The terms used throughout the Compact shall have the meaning set forth below:

   a. **ADPH Patient Transfer Center**–The Alabama Department of Public Health, along with coordinating representatives from the Alabama Hospital Association and other organizations representing entities providing patient care, will staff a patient transfer center during a public health emergency or mass casualty disaster. The purpose of this center will be to coordinate efforts between hospitals and other health care entities and the State Emergency Operations Center to ensure appropriate transfer of patients and optimum utilization of health care resources within the State. The primary tool for assessing the availability of health care resources and coordinating transfers will be the AIMS system.

   b. **"Affected Entity"** is a Participating Entity which is impacted by a Disaster.

   c. **"AIMS,"** the Alabama Incident Management System, is a computer software program that allows the Alabama Department of Public Health to monitor the resources of hospitals, nursing homes, community health centers, and ambulance companies during times of disasters.

d. **"Assisting Entity"** is a Participating Entity party which is available upon request to assist an Affected Entity.

e. **"Designated Representative"** is the individual or position designated by each Participating Entity to act as a liaison with ADPH during any revisions of the Operating Procedures and to communicate with the Affected Entity and the appropriate individuals within the representative's own healthcare organization in the event of a Disaster.

f. **"Disaster"** means a major incident occurring or imminent within a Participating Entity and/or in the surrounding community, that overwhelms its ability to function as a health care delivery organization and typically requires the notification of the State emergency management agency, local emergency response agencies, and the responsible Public Health Department. However, activation of the Mutual Aid Compact is not dependent upon the proclamation of a State of Emergency by the Governor of the State of Alabama under Chapter 16 of Title 31 of the Code of Ala.1975. Disasters include, but are not limited to, natural disasters, such as hurricanes, and man-made disasters, such as acts of terrorism. A Disaster may affect the entire facility or only a portion of the facility or its health care staff.

g. **"Evacuation"** means the process of moving patients and staff from the Affected Entity due to a disaster that threatens life and/or the ability of the Affected Entity to provide health care services.

h. **"Operating Procedures"** means the system for implementing this Compact which includes, but is not limited to, the following: (i) a method for making and responding to requests for the transfer of patients and/or the sharing of staff, equipment, supplies and other essential services; (ii) an agreed-upon technology to facilitate communication between the parties in the event of a Disaster or Evacuation; (iii) the role of State, Federal and other aid agencies in the event of a Disaster; (iv) the steps required when an Affected Entity and/or an entire region experience a Disaster (v) the development and/or designation of Public Health disease surveillance activities and systems for timely notification of hospital capacity status; cases or suspect cases of diseases; unusual outbreaks which may be associated with a terrorist attack; and identification of credentialing, licensure, medical staff, and liability issues.

i. **"Other Entity"** any entity in a contiguous State that signs a similar Compact compatible herewith.

j. **"Other Health Care Entity"** is any health care organization such as community health center, Indian Health Services clinic, physician practice group, medical needs shelter, ADPH-licensed EMS service provider, rescue squad, or mental health hospital or clinic or ADPH licensed nursing home that has joined the Compact by signing this agreement.

k. **"Participating Entity"** any Alabama entity/health system agency, entity, or organization that transfers, or receives patients, or provides health or medical care or supplies or equipment, or any participating entity in a contiguous State that signs a similar compact compatible herewith or any "Other Health Care Entity." This can include, but is not limited to: in-patient facilities such as general or specialty hospitals; nursing homes; federally qualified health care centers and other such clinics or health care centers; and emergency medical service providers whether private or government owned.

l. **"State ADPH Coordinator** is the individual designated by ADPH as the person with whom participating entities shall coordinate during an event.

ARTICLE II

OPERATING PROCEDURES

2.1 Participating Entities agree to identify a Designated Representative (liaison) and at least two back-up individuals to participate in revisions, when needed, of Operating Procedures, attached as Exhibit B. The names and contact information for the Participating Entity's Designated Representative, back-up individuals, and other key personnel are attached hereto as Exhibit A. Participating Entities agree to provide ADPH with timely updates (see Exhibit A) where available via AIMS.

2.2 The Designated Representative and/or back-up individuals shall attend meetings and conferences scheduled by ADPH through the ADPH Center for Emergency Preparedness to discuss issues related to this Compact and if needed, to revise the Operating Procedures. The Designated Representative shall act as a liaison with representatives of the ADPH Patient Transfer Center and the Affected Entity, in the event of a Disaster.

2.3 In the event of any inconsistency between this Compact and the finalized Operating Procedures, the terms of the Operating Procedures shall govern.

2.4 The Participating Entities agree to participate as appropriate, in Public Health disease surveillance activities and systems for timely notification of entity capacity status, as set forth in the Operating Procedures.

ARTICLE III

COMMUNICATION BETWEEN PARTICIPATING ENTITIES DURING A DISASTER

3.1 In the event of a Disaster, the Participating Entities agree to:

   a. Communicate and coordinate their response efforts via their Designated Representatives (Liaisons) in accordance with this Compact and the Operating Procedures;

   b. Logon to and activate the ability to receive and send information via AIMS, if available, and to maintain such capability for the duration of the event.

   c. Communicate, including receiving alert information, in accordance with the Operating Procedures, by phone, fax, AIMS and/or email, 800 MHz radio, HAM radio, or other means of communication, and to maintain radio capability to communicate as a minimum back-up.

ARTICLE IV

TRANSFERS

4.1 Requirements regarding transferring and receiving patients apply only to Participating Entities that are inpatient facilities. Other types of parties will comply to the extent of their capability in the patient transfer process. The Participating Entities agree to accept patients transferred by any Affected Entity under the terms and conditions set forth in this Compact and in accordance with the Operating Procedures.

4.2 The Participating Entities agree that in transferring patients from an Affected Entity to an Assisting Entity, the Affected Entity shall contact the ADPH Patient Transfer Center as soon as possible and shall enter the pertinent information regarding the transfer in AIMS. If the Affected Entity cannot find an Assisting Entity, it may request help from the ADPH Patient Transfer Center in doing so.

4.3 The Participating Entities agree that in accepting the transfer of patients from the Affected Entity, the Assisting Entity will make reasonable efforts, whenever feasible, to:

   a. Communicate with the Affected Entity regarding the numbers and types/acuity of patients who may be transferred. This communication may be via any communications system available including AIMS or any successor system.

b. Accept all transfers from Affected Entity that are within the limitations communicated by the Designated Representative. Assisting Entity shall not be obligated to accept any patients that exceed its ability to assist herein, its capacity or its staffing, which shall be determined at the Assisting Entity's sole discretion.

4.4 The Participating Entities agree to cooperate with each other in billing and collecting for services furnished to patients pursuant to this Compact and the Operating Procedures attached hereto.

ARTICLE V

STAFF, SUPPLIES, AND EQUIPMENT

5.1 The Participating Entities agree, in the event of a Disaster, to use reasonable efforts to make clinical staff, medical and general supplies, including pharmaceuticals, and biomedical equipment (including, but not limited to ventilators, monitors, and infusion pumps) available to each other in accordance with the Operating Procedures. Each Participating Entity shall be entitled to use its reasonable judgment regarding the type and amount of staff, supplies, and equipment it can provide without adversely affecting its own ability to provide services.

5.2 The Participating Entities agree to cooperate with each other to determine appropriate compensation for the use of staff, and for supplies and equipment shared in accordance with the Operating Procedures.

ARTICLE VI

NON-EMPLOYED MEDICAL STAFF

6.1 In the event of a Disaster, the Participating Entities agree to inform their non-employee medical staff members of any requests for assistance and offer them the opportunity to volunteer their professional services. The Participating Entities shall cooperate with each other to provide in a timely manner the information necessary to verify employment status, licensure, training, and other information necessary in order for such volunteers to receive emergency credentials.

ARTICLE VII

MISCELLANEOUS PROVISIONS

7.1 This Compact, together with the attached exhibits, constitutes the entire compact between the Participating Entities.

7.2 Amendments to this Compact must be in writing and signed by the Participating Entities.

7.3 Nothing in this compact shall be construed as limiting the rights of the Participating Entities to affiliate or contract with any other entity operating an entity or other health care facility on either a limited or general basis while this compact is in effect. This Compact is not intended to supersede such agreements; neither is this Compact intended to establish a preferred status for patients of any Affected Entity.

7.4 A Participating Entity may at anytime terminate its participation in the Compact by providing sixty-day written notice to the ADPH Center for Emergency Preparedness. However, if no such notice is given, the Compact remains in effect in perpetuity.

7.5 In the event that the Governor of the State of Alabama has proclaimed a State of Emergency, all parties as entities and all individuals performing any functions within the scope and line of their duties for or on behalf of any such party, performing functions under the terms of this Compact are recognized by ADPH as exercising the governmental powers and functions of the State of Alabama and are considered by ADPH as emergency management workers or entities providing resources to the State of Alabama as appropriate in fulfillment of immunity provisions of Chapter 16 of Title 31 of the Code of Ala. 1975.

7.6 Any notices required or permitted hereunder shall be sufficiently given and deemed received upon personal delivery, or upon the third business day following deposit in the U.S. Mail, if sent by registered or certified mail, postage prepaid, addressed, or delivered as follows:

Copies to:

Participating Entity: _____
Street Address: _____
City/State/Zip: _____

Alabama Department of Public Health
Center for Emergency Preparedness
RSA Tower, Suite 1310 Montgomery, Alabama 36130-3017

EDITOR'S NOTE: *Signature page and Exhibit A-Agency listing were deleted.*

EXHIBIT B

This Exhibit is intended to append to the ADPH Approved Mutual Aid Compact between the parties to such Compact (The Compact) and to basically serve as a guideline for the implementation of the compact, with the understanding that the terms set forth herein may not be applicable in all situations. The terminology found in this appendix is defined in the Compact.

1.00 Patient and Patient Transfer Responsibilities

Each Participating Entity, as appropriate, is willing to accept patients transferred by the other party under the terms and conditions set forth in this Exhibit and as coordinated through AIMS. Terms in this Exhibit are only applicable in the event the transfer of patients cannot be handled by the Participating Entity through local efforts.

1.1 **Initiation of transfer.** Only the Administrator or a designee from each Affected Entity has the authority to initiate the evacuation, transfer, or receipt of personnel, material resources/supplies, or patients. If evacuation of patients is needed, and the Participating Entity does not have an agreement with an Assisting Entity to handle incoming patients, the administrator or designee of the Affected Entity will notify local EMA and ADPH Patient Transfer Center through AIMS. After EMA/ADPH instruction, the Affected Entity will notify emergency medical services of needed assistance in handling transfers. It is assumed in disasters that affected entities are already working closely with local public health and disaster/emergency services.

1.2 **Documentation:** The Affected Entity and Assisting Entity are responsible where practical for tracking the destination of all patients transferred through AIMS.

1.3 **Transfer Responsibilities of Affected Entity.** The parties agree that in the event it becomes necessary to transfer patients from the Affected Entity to the Assisting Entity, the Affected Entity shall after initial contact:

   a. Contact the Designated Representative at the Assisting Entity as soon as the Affected Entity becomes aware of the need to transfer patients. The request for the transfer of patients initially can be made verbally. However, it must be followed up with a written communication where practical prior to the actual transferring of any patients;

   b. Provide the number of patients needing to be transferred;

c. Comply with any limitations communicated to the Affected Entity regarding the numbers and types/acuity of patients that the Assisting Entity is able to accept;

d. Identify type of specialized services required (e.g., ICU, ventilator, etc.). To the extent practical and available, the Affected Entity is responsible for sending extraordinary drugs or other special patient needs (e.g., specialized equipment, blood products) along with the patient, if requested by the Assisting Entity.

e. Triage all patients prior to transfer to verify that the types and acuity of services required are within the scope of services the Assisting Entity is able to provide;

f. Arrange for the transport of each patient to the Assisting Entity, with the support of such medical personnel and equipment as is required by the patient's condition. The Affected Entity is responsible for coordinating and financing the transportation of patients to the receiving facility and tracking costs related to transport;

g. Once admitted, transferred patient(s) become the patient(s) of and are under care of the Assisting Entity's medical practitioner until discharged, transferred or reassigned;

h. Deliver where practical to the Assisting Entity, with each patient transferred, medical Records, or copies thereof, sufficient to indicate the patient's diagnoses, condition, and treatment provided and planned; and

i. If feasible, inventory the patient's personal effects and valuables transported with the patient to the Assisting Entity. The Affected Entity shall deliver the inventory and the patient's valuables to the personnel transporting the patient, and receive a receipt for such items from the Assisting Entity.

1.4 **Transfer Responsibilities of Assisting Entity.** The parties agree that in accepting the transfer of patients from the Affected Entity, the Assisting Entity shall:

a. Have an Administrator or Designated Representative available 24 hours a day, 7 days a week to implement this Compact and to communicate with the Affected Entity regarding the numbers and types/acuity of patients who may be transferred.

b. Accept all transfers from the Administrator or Affected Entity that are within the limitations communicated by the Designated Representative of the Assisting Entity. The Assisting Entity shall not be obligated to accept any patients which exceed its ability to assist herein, its capacity or staffing, which shall be determined in the Assisting Entity's sole discretion.

c. Record in the clinical records of each transferred patient notations of the condition of the patient upon arrival at the Assisting Entity.

d. If personal effects and valuables of the patient are transported with the patient, check those items against the inventory prepared by the Affected Entity, and issue a receipt for such items as are received by the Assisting Entity to the personnel transporting the patient.

e. Designate, upon arrival or as soon as practical, the admitting service and an admitting medical practitioner for each transferred patient.

1.5 Discharge of Patients. If a transferred patient is discharged by the Assisting Entity, the Assisting Entity will return to the Affected Entity any original medical records, including x-ray films, transferred with the patient. If the Affected Entity is not then able to receive the returned medical records, the Assisting Entity will retain the records in the Assisting Entity's records department until requested by the Affected Entity.

1.6 Charges for Services. All charges for services provided at the Affected Entity or at the Assisting Entity for patients transferred pursuant to this Compact shall be collected by the party providing such services directly from the patient, third party payer or other source normally billed by the party. The parties agree to cooperate with each other in billing and collecting for services furnished to patients pursuant to this Compact. The billing and collection of charges for transportation of the patient from the Affected Entity to the Assisting Entity (and to return the patient to the Affected Entity) shall be the responsibility of the Affected Entity, and the transporting medium.

1.7 Notifications. In routing patients from an Affected Entity to an Assisting Entity, and in accordance with all applicable State and Federal laws and regulations, the Affected Entity may inform ADPH and other appropriate governmental agency(ies) as soon as they are aware of the need to transfer patients, informing the agency(ies) of the number of patients needing transfer, the type of care they will require, and their acuity level. The Affected Entity is also responsible where practical for notifying both the patient's family or guardian and the patient's attending or personal physician of the situation. The Assisting Entity may assist in notifying the patient's family and personal physician.

2.00 Supplies, Equipment and Pharmaceuticals

Each party agrees to use its commercially reasonable efforts to make general and medical equipment and supplies (i.e., infusion pumps, pharmaceuticals, monitors, ventilators, laboratory supplies) available to each other under this Exhibit in the event of a disaster, upon request. Supplies may be requested to address the needs of transferred patients or may be requested to address disasters that require additional supplies without movement of patients. The Assisting Entity shall be entitled to use its own reasonable judgment regarding the type and amount of supplies that it can provide. The Affected Entity that receives the supplies will reimburse the Assisting Entity based on the actual cost of those supplies as herein below specified.

2.1 **Equipment.** Each party agrees to use commercially reasonable efforts to make biomedical equipment, including, but not limited to ventilators, monitors and infusion pumps, available to an Affected Entity in the event of a disaster, upon request. The Assisting Entity shall be entitled to use its own reasonable judgment regarding the equipment that it can provide without adversely affecting its own ability to provide services.

2.2 **Communication of Request.** Initial communications of need shall be made through the local EMA, ADPH and, then to the Assisting Entity in accordance with EMA guidelines. Affected Entity's request to Assisting Entities for transfer of supplies or equipment initially may be made verbally. The request, however, must be followed up with written communication such as HEICS 201. The written request must be submitted to the Assisting Entity prior to the receipt of any material resources at the Affected Entity. The Affected Entity will identify to the Assisting Entity the following:

a. Indicate the quantity and exact type of resources;

b. Estimate how quickly the request must be filled;

c. Note the time period for which the resources will be needed; and

d. Specify the location where the resources should be delivered.

2.3 **Supply of Equipment and Supplies.** The Assisting Entity will supply a copy of its standard accounting record such as HEICS Form 3-10 and other required copies of paperwork to the Affected Entity for all equipment loaned. The Assisting Entity will identify how long it will take it to fill the requests, as rapid response is a key component.

2.4 **Documentation.** Parties have an obligation to document the quantity and condition of any equipment and supplies that are exchanged during a disaster. Both parties to a transaction should be able to document the quantity and condition of equipment loaned, the receipt and return (including condition) of any equipment.

2.5 **Supervision.** The Affected Entity is responsible for appropriate use and maintenance of all borrowed supplies or equipment.

2.6 **Transportation.** When feasible, the Affected Entity will be responsible for transporting the loaned equipment. If the Affected Entity is unable to transport the Equipment, the Assisting Entity will arrange for shipping/ transportation of the loaned equipment to and from the Affected Entity. All expenses of shipping/transport shall be the responsibility of the Affected Entity.

2.7 **Risk of Loss.** The Affected Entity assumes the risk of loss or damage to equipment while in its possession or in transit. The Affected Entity will promptly notify the Assisting Entity if damage or loss of equipment occurs.

2.8 **Return of Equipment.** The Affected Entity shall use reasonable care under the circumstances in the operation and control of all materials and supplies used by them during the period of assistance. Unused supplies may be returned, provided that they are unopened and in good and usable condition. The Affected Entity will promptly return equipment to the Assisting Entity upon request, unless return of the equipment would be life-threatening to a patient at the Affected Entity or would otherwise significantly compromise the health or safety of a patient. If return of equipment is not feasible, arrangements for compensation will be made between the entities as herein below specified.

2.9 **Compensation.** Entities operating under a signed mutual aid compact may receive reimbursement to cover their expenses should such reimbursement become available.

2.10 **Repair and Maintenance of Equipment.** The Affected Entity shall pay for all repairs to borrowed equipment as determined necessary by its on-site supervisor(s) to maintain such equipment in safe and operational condition.

3.00 Personnel

The Administrator or designee of an Affected Entity as assisted if necessary by the Medical Staff Director, in conjunction with the departmental directors of affected services, will make a determination as to whether medical staff and other personnel will be needed at their facility. Personnel may be out-stationed or dispatched as herein below specified. While providing services to the Affected Entity, employees of the Assisting Entity shall remain as employees of their respective Entity while responding to, or performing an emergency mutual aid function hereunder and until which time the employee is relieved of further emergency mutual aid responsibility by a duly authorized official.

3.1 **Requesting Procedure.** The Affected Entity requests personnel by notifying the local EMA and ADPH via AIMS and subsequently the Assisting Entity of a need for assistance, in accordance with EMA guidelines. After EMA/ADPH instruction, the Administrator or designee of the Affected Entity will coordinate directly with the Administrator or designee of the Assisting Entity for this assistance. The request for the transfer of personnel made by the Affected Entity may initially be made verbally. The request, however, must be followed up with written documentation. This should occur prior to the arrival of personnel at the Affected Entity. The Affected Entity will specify the following to the donor facility:

 a. Type and number of personnel needed;

 b. Estimate of how quickly the resources are needed;

 c. Location where they are to report; and

 d. Estimate of how long the personnel will be needed.

3.2 **Credentialing of Physician Personnel.** All party entities will put into place in their entity policies provisions compliant with JCAHO, or CMS as appropriate, requirements for temporary credentialing or privileging of received physician personnel as dispatched by Assisting Entities.

3.3 **Dispatching Volunteer Personnel.** Hospital Volunteer Personnel dispatched from Assisting Entities should be limited to staff that are fully accredited or credentialed in the Assisting Entity. No resident physicians, medical/nursing students, or in-training persons will be volunteered by the Assisting Entity. If in-training persons wish to volunteer directly to the affected facility, they may do so, through ADPH Volunteer Network. They could also volunteer to work at alternate care or triage sites.

3.4 **Receiving of volunteer personnel.** The Affected Entity will accept the professional licenses, credentialing and approval of Assisting Entities in compliance with this Exhibit. The Affected Entity will be responsible for the following:

 a. Meet the arriving personnel (usually done by Affected Entity's security department or another designated employee);

 b. Ask arriving personnel to present their Entity identification at the site designated by the Affected Entity's emergency command center;

 c. Copy or scan the person's identification card to verify the volunteer's status and keep same in an appropriate file for location or audit purposes.

3.5 **Supervision of Personnel by Affected Entity.** The Affected Entity's Administrator or designee identifies where and to whom the dispatched personnel should report. Professional staff from the Affected Entity shall be assigned to supervise volunteer personnel. The supervisor will meet with dispatched professionals as soon as possible after arrival and brief them of the incident status and their assignments. The emergency staffing rules of the Affected Entity will govern assigned shifts.

3.6 **Housing/Meals:** The Affected Entity is responsible for securing housing and meals for volunteer healthcare personnel sent by Assisting Entity.

3.7 **Financial Responsibilities and Payments to Dispatched Staff.** Dispatched professional staff shall continue to be employees of their dispatching institution and received salary and benefits, employee pensions and other benefits, and worker's compensation insurance from the dispatching facility; however, the Affected Entity will reimburse the Assisting Entity for all such costs related to dispatched staff. These costs include receiving wages and benefits from their Assisting Entity as the donated personnel would normally receive, including shift differentials and overtime pay. Costs also include the pro-rata share of worker's compensation coverage premiums as determined by Generally Accepted Accounting Principles (GAAP). The Affected Entity will reimburse the Assisting Entity within 90 days following receipt of the invoice.

3.8 **Non-Employed Medical Staff.** The Assisting Hospital shall inform its non-employee medical staff members of the request for assistance and offer them the opportunity to participate in the Assisting Hospital's response as is appropriate in the judgment of the Assisting Hospital. The Assisting Hospital shall cooperate with the Affected Hospital to provide promptly the information necessary to verify employment status, licensure and training necessary to perform the procedures requiring assistance of volunteer non-employee medical staff members. To the extent necessary or desirable, the Assisting Hospital will provide the Affected Hospital with copies of the relevant medical staff credentialing files to support the grant of emergency staff privileges.

3.9 **Patient Care Staff.** The parties agree to use their commercially reasonable efforts to make clinical staff available to an Affected Entity in the event of a disaster, upon request. The Assisting Entity shall be entitled to use its own reasonable judgment regarding the clinical staff it can provide without adversely affecting its own ability to provide services. Clinical staff subject to this Compact shall be limited to staff employed by the Assisting Entity except that Non-Employed Medical Staff may be considered as employed for these purposes.

3.10 Responsibility for Personnel. The parties agree that the personnel made available to the Affected Entity shall be under the supervision and control of the Affected Entity while performing any actions in response to the Affected Entity's request for personnel.

3.11 Personnel Files. The Assisting Entity shall, upon request, provide to the Affected Entity copies of personnel files sufficient to document the licensure, training and competence of the dispatched staff. The Assisting Entity shall use its commercially reasonable efforts to ensure that such records comply with licensure and accreditation requirements applicable to the Assisting Entity.

3.12 Recall of Staff. The Assisting Entity may recall its clinical staff at any time within its sole discretion. Parties will make every effort to provide adequate notice so as to allow the Affected Entity to arrange staffing from other facilities or agencies.

3.13 Non-Dispatched Volunteer Personnel. Volunteers who are not dispatched by an Assisting Entity will not be reimbursed for labor performed while participating under this Compact, nor may Assisting Entities claim reimbursement for such.

4.00 Ancillary Services

4.1 Ancillary Services. The parties agree to use their commercially reasonable efforts to make essential ancillary services, including, but not limited to, clinical laboratory and dietary services, available to an Affected Entity in the event of a disaster, upon request. When feasible, the Affected Entity will be responsible for all transportation and delivery services associated with the ancillary services, such as the delivery of laboratory specimens and the pick up and delivery of dietary supplies. If the Affected Entity is unable to provide transportation/delivery, the Assisting Entity will arrange for transportation/delivery to and from the Affected Entity. All expenses of shipping/transport shall be the responsibility of the Affected Entity. The Affected Entity will compensate the Assisting Entity at cost to the Assisting Entity.

5.00 Liability and Insurance

Each party shall throughout the term of the Compact to which the Exhibit is appended, maintain comprehensive general liability insurance, workers' compensation insurance, property insurance, professional liability (malpractice) insurance, and other insurances as required by the laws of the State of Alabama or by Federal law as herein below specified. General and professional liability insurance coverage shall be maintained in the minimum amount of $1,000,000.00 per occurrence and $3,000,000.00 annual aggregate. Upon request, parties shall provide to the other party certificates evidencing the existence of such insurance coverage. Each party may at its option satisfy its obligations under this section through self-insurance programs and protections deemed by it to be comparable to the insurance coverage described herein, and upon request, provide to the other party information showing that the self-insurance programs offer such comparable protection.

5.1 Workers' Compensation, Liability, and Directors' and Officers' Coverage.

    a. Worker's Compensation Coverage. Each party is responsible for complying with the State of Alabama's Workers' Compensation Act. Each party should understand that workers' compensation coverage does not automatically extend to volunteers.

    b. Automobile Liability Coverage: Each party is responsible for insuring that it is in compliance with the State of Alabama's motor vehicle financial responsibility laws.

    c. Director's and Officers' Coverage. Each party agrees to have in force or obtain director's and officers' liability coverage.

6.00 Relationship of Parties

6.1 Relationship of Parties to Each Other. None of the provisions of the Compact to which this Exhibit is appended are intended to create nor shall be deemed or construed to create a partnership, joint venture, employee/employer relationship or any relationship between the parties, other than that of independent entities contracting with each other hereunder solely for the purpose of effecting the provisions of this Compact.

6.2 **Relationship to the State of Alabama.** It is the intent of the Compact to which this Exhibit is appended that when the Governor of the State of Alabama has proclaimed a State of emergency for the purposes of Title 31, *Code of Alabama* 1975, the parties hereto when performing pursuant to such proclamation, are to be considered to the extent allowable by law as performing State or State-directed functions under '31-9-17, *Code of Ala.* 1975 and should be entitled to immunities granted under that Section. Likewise, the officers, agents, servants and employees of parties when performing under such a proclaimed State of emergency should be considered "emergency management workers" as defined by '31-9-16, *Code of Ala.* 1975 and should be entitled to immunities granted under that Section.

6.3 **Department's Role in Coordinating Governmental Reimbursement.** Nothing in this Compact or the Attachments to it is to be construed as being contingent upon the availability or reimbursement of funds from any Federal source and the parties herein shall fully comply with the terms herein without regard to such reimbursement issues. To the extent that Title 31 has been invoked and reimbursement is available from any governmental or other private sources other than as herein above provided, the Department will serve as a facilitator and coordinator for the collection and proper routing of reimbursement funds.

6.4 **Relationships with and Affiliation with Other Facilities.** Nothing in the Compact to which this Exhibit is appended shall be construed as limiting the right of the parties to affiliate or contract with any other entity operating an entity or other health care facility on either a limited or general basis while the Compact is in effect. Each party acknowledges that, in the event of a large scale disaster, the ability of the Assisting Entity to accept patients from the Affected Entity will be affected by the receipt of patients from other sources, including direct admissions from the community, transfers of patients from other facilities, or patient assignment through NDMS. The Compact to which this Exhibit is appended is not intended to establish a preferred status for patients of the Affected Entities. All decisions regarding allocation of available facilities will be made by the Assisting Entity using its best judgment about the needs of its community.

6.5 **Relationship to the Public.** Each facility is responsible for developing and co-ordinating internally, and locally, with appropriate organizations, especially the media, on how each party will coordinate communication in a disaster. A Joint Information Center (JIC) is an ideal structure for coordinating information releases. Designating a Public Information Officer (PIO) in each facility helps coordinate communication via the JIC to the public. PIOs normally work with Command Staff to develop a facility response to cover its most likely events. Parties are encouraged to have their PIO work with other party PIOs to familiarize one another with each other's protocols for addressing the media, and to practice JIC to JIC coordination.

6.6 Relationship to NDMS. Nothing in the Compact to which this Exhibit is appended is intended to in any way supersede or interfere with standing Compacts that any of the parties may have with the National Disaster Medical System (NDMS.) However, it is expected that in a disaster, the State Health Officer or representatives from the Patient Transfer Center will be in constant contact with the State's NDMS representative to ensure optimal coordination of Statewide health care services and the best use of available health system resources.

6.7 Assignment. This Compact and the rights of the parties hereunder, may not be assigned by any party, without the prior written consent of the other parties.

6.8 No Waiver. No waiver of a breach of any provision of this Compact shall be construed to be a waiver of any breach of any other provision of this Compact or of any succeeding breach of the same provision.

6.9 Relationship to the Public in General. The execution of this Compact shall not give rise to any liability or responsibility for failure to respond to any request for assistance, lack of speed in answering such a request, inadequacy of equipment, or abilities of the responding personnel.

7.00 Mobilization and Demobilization Procedures

7.1 Mobilization Plan. Each party shall develop and update on a regular basis a plan providing for the effective mobilization of its resources and facilities.

7.2 Demobilization. Parties hereto will provide and coordinate any necessary demobilization procedures and post-event stress debriefing.

ANNEX II: Sample Mass Gathering Event Planning Tools

Introduction
The following sample documentation is intended to provide one possible method for documenting the planning and response to a mass gathering incident.

Use of Fictional Location: "Townville"
Townville is a fictional city used for illustrative purposes. Names of past Presidents of the United States were used to illustrate key positions within the Incident Command System (ICS). Any similarity to an actual city or location is coincidental.

Demographics of "Townville"
Townville is a city covering 60 square miles and home to over 200,000 residents. The median income for a family is just under $40,000 annually. Per capita income is just over $20,000. A breakdown of population age groups can be seen in the table below.

Age	Percent Population
<18	22%
18 to 24	13%
25 to 44	32%
45 to 64	20%
65+	11%

Townville is home to 5 different Fortune 500 companies, a half dozen medium-sized sports venues including a 13,000 seat baseball park and a 12,000 seat multipurpose arena. A large public university occupies much of the city's downtown real estate. A much smaller private university also resides in Townville. There are three high schools and a dozen middle and elementary schools within the city.

Townville is home to a level-one trauma center and two other medium-sized hospitals with specialties in stroke and cardiology. Four other hospitals are within easy reach of the city's Emergency Medical Services (EMS). There are six nursing homes and numerous group homes within the city.

EMS in Townville is supported by 18 full-time Advanced Life Support (ALS) ambulances and 2 ALS nonsupervisor nontransport units, and 12 Basic Life Support (BLS) first responder engine companies. Mutual aid EMS is provided by 3 adjoining municipalities in Wayne County with a total of 14 ALS and 24 BLS ambulances.

This page was intentionally left blank.

Sample EMS Operations Plan

Townville Marathon
September 29, 2011

Table of Contents

Event Background 114
Potential Impact 114
Key Contact Information 115
Command Structure 116
Resource Listing 117
Personnel Rehabilitation 117
Course Treatment Facilities 117
Mutual Aid Response 118
Communications 118
MCI Response 120
MEDEVACs 120
Other Contingencies 120

Event Background

The Townville Marathon will take place on September 29, 2011. The event actually includes the following races: the Shriners 8k Race, Whole Foods Half Marathon, and the 1st National Townville Marathon.

Duration: The first race (8k) will begin at 0700, the half marathon will begin at 0730, and the full marathon will begin at 0800. Projected completion time is 1500 hours. Runners are limited to a 7-hour maximum.

Course: The course is a 26.2-mile race, covering most of the city. The start line is at 12th and Broad, and the finish line is at 1st and Main.

Expected Attendance: There are 15,000 people registered as participants, and 20,000 spectators are possible.

Weather Forecast: It is predicted to be partly cloudy, high of 68 °F, low of 36 °F with a 20 percent chance of precipitation (as of 9-20-11).

Sponsoring Organization: The organization sponsoring the event is the Townville Sports Group, located at 1234 Presidents Avenue, Townville, MI 48125. Their main phone number is 313-123-4567.

Potential Impact

The most significant impact will be on EMS at the event itself. There are 15,000 potential participants of widely varying levels of fitness competing in a 5.0, 13.1, and 26.2-mile running race, combined with 20,000 possible spectators. Based on last year's event data, 0.8 percent of all participants sought medical attention. If this ratio holds true this year, onsite medical services could experience 123 or more medical requests and 9 EMS transports from the event.

EMS operations outside of the actual event will also be impacted. Travel throughout the city will be impeded for 7 hours or more during the busiest part of the day. Communication officers and field units alike must plan for this and route accordingly.

Key Contact Information

Emergency Medical Services	
Townville EMS (TEMS) Agency	**Townville Fire Department (TFD)**
EMS Communications (XXX) XXX-XXXX Capt. James Polk (Unit 100) EMS Operations (Unified Command) (XXX) XXX-XXXX Sgt. Martin Buren Bike Team Leader (XXX)-XXX-XXXX	FD Communications (XXX) XXX-XXXX Battalion Chief Chester Arthur EMS Operations (Unified Command) (XXX) XXX-XXXX
Townville Police Department (TPD)	**Sports Group**
PD Communications (XXX) XXX-XXXX Lt. Warren Harding (Unified Command) (XXX) XXX-XXXX	John Tyler (Unified Command) (XXX) XXX-XXXX James Buchanan (XXX) XXX-XXXX
Mass Casualty Incident (MCI) Resources	**Aeromedical Resources**
State EOC (XXX) XXX-XXXX Townville Medical Center MCI Line (XXX) XXX-XXXX Wayne County Communications (XXX) XXX-XXXX Monroe County Communications (XXX) XXX-XXXX	Townville Medflight (XXX) XXX-XXXX Townville Life Flight (XXX) XXX-XXXX

Command Structure

The following initial command structure will be in place for the event. This structure may be expanded as necessary in accordance with ICS principles.

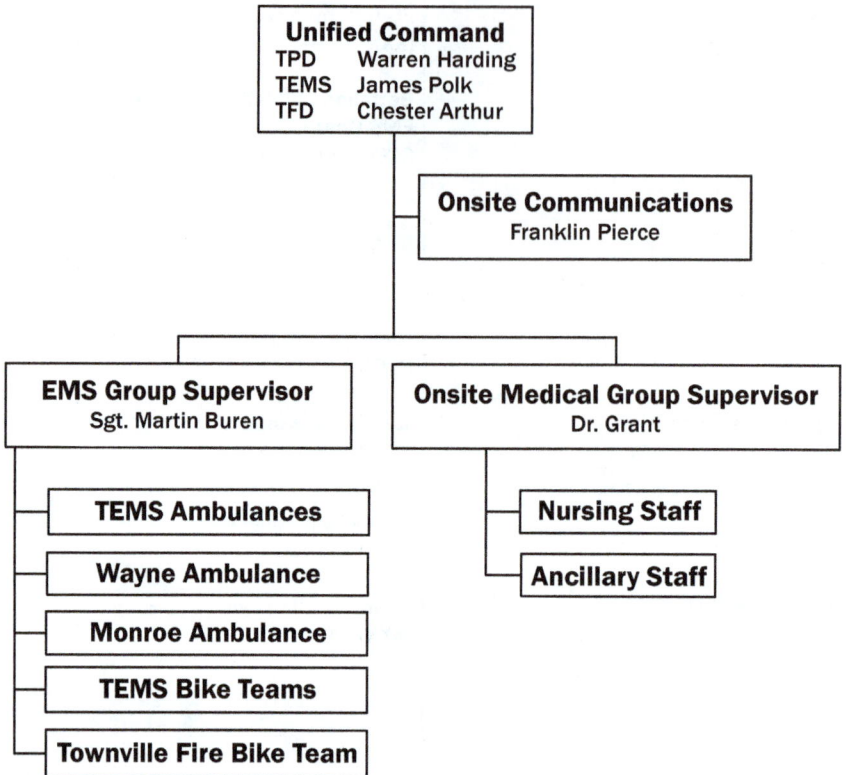

Resource Listing

The following EMS resources will be available on scene:

Personnel	Vehicles	Equipment/Supplies
TEMS Communication: 1	ALS Ambulance: 5	**In Type II ambulance:** 1 extra stretcher
TEMS BLS: 6	ALS Bike Team: 3	2 extra drug boxes
TEMS ALS: 6	BLS Bike Team: 1	2 extra jump kits
TFD BLS: 2	Type II ambulance: 1 (As a logistics support vehicle)	2 extra Reeves sleeves 1 extra ECG monitor
Monroe ALS: 2	Unit 30 (in quarters)	Extra blankets
Monroe BLS: 1	MCI-1 at TEMS HQ	Extra towels
Wayne ALS: 2	Resource 2 at TEMS HQ	Command laptop and binder 6 portable oxygen tanks 6 oxygen regulators
Physicians: 2	Ancillary staff: Unknown	2 spare UHF radios
Nurses: 5-7		1 spare 800 MHz radio Large cooler with ice 3 cases IV fluids

Personnel Rehabilitation

Each TEMS ambulance will carry extra water and sports drinks for bike teams. Rehabilitation for EMS personnel will also be available at multiple points along the course. Designated rehabilitation areas are as follows:

- Public parking area at 10th and Main.

- Mile 6 water stop near Grover Avenue and Massachusetts Road.

- Mile 12 water stop near Tower Drive and Huntington Avenue.

- Mile 20 water stop near Forest Avenue and Henry Road.

Course Treatment Facilities

Two course treatment facilities will be available. The primary medical treatment facility is located at 20th and Main in a parking garage on the NE corner. This facility will be equipped with 45 cots, IV therapy supplies, oxygen, and basic medical supplies. This facility will be staffed by a sports medicine physician (Dr. Grant), several Registered Nurses (RNs), and additional ancillary staff.

The secondary treatment facility will be located at Forest Avenue and Tree Road (Marathon mile 21/Half Marathon mile 8). This facility will be very minimally equipped with a single physician, an RN, and a sports trainer.

Mutual Aid Response

Prior to the race, surrounding jurisdictions have been polled as to what mutual aid resources will be available if the need arises. Resources available include:

Wayne County
ALS Ambulances: 4
BLS Ambulances: 2
EMS Officers: 1
Support Units: 0

Monroe County
ALS Ambulances: 6
BLS Ambulances: 4
EMS Officers: 2
Support Units: 1

Transit Authority
Buses: 6

Any responding mutual aid units will provide care according to their own approved local protocols. Communications will be handled by field communications on site on predetermined talk-groups.

Communications

Onsite EMS communications will be handled over our standard ultrahigh frequency (UHF) radio system, with the 800 MHz system as a backup. Communications between field communications and the TEMS communication center will be handled by cellular phone and over the UHF radio system. Communications between event staff and EMS will be handled over their UHF radio system. Primary zones and channels are outlined below.

Use	System	Zone	Channel/Frequency
Event EMS Communications	UHF	N/A	TEMS EMS 3 or TEMSPD on 800 MHz system
Mutual Aid EMS Communications	800 MHz	1	3 (TAC 1)
Field Comm to Comm Center	UHF	N/A	2 (TEMS EMS 2)
Field to Incoming TEMS Units	UHF	N/A	3 (TEMS EMS 3)
Event Staff to EMS	UHF	N/A	2 (SB Medcomm)
Field Comm to Hospital (MCI Plan)	UHF	N/A	14 (MED 9)
Field Comm to Medevac	VHF	N/A	155.205 (EMS Statewide)

Call taking and response plans are outlined below:

For calls received from standby units at the event or event staff:

Units staffing the event are to report all patients to field communications. Units calling in patient contacts need to report:

- Location;
- Bib Number;
- Complaint;
- Triage Status (Red, Yellow, Green); and
- Need for transport unit.

If no transport is needed, field communications will keep track of the incident and times for later quality assurance (QA)/quality improvement (QI). No involvement with the communications center is needed.

If the unit on scene determines a transport unit is needed, the field communications officer will report the location, unit on scene, and priority of the incident to the communications center over EMS channel 2. Priority will be determined as follows:

- Red Triage Status = Priority 1;
- Yellow Triage Status = Priority 2; and
- Green Triage Status = Priority 3.

Field communications will also advise the communications center of an evacuation point for the transport unit to respond to. The communications center will then dispatch a unit to the evacuation point based on the priority advised by field communications. Both the responding ambulance and the standby unit on scene will be logged to the call for timekeeping purposes.

If the incident is called in by the event staff, field communications will dispatch the closest standby unit to the incident; it is at the field communications officer's discretion whether or not a transport unit is initially dispatched. If a transport unit is needed, dispatch procedures outlined above will be used.

For calls received by 9-1-1 line from the event:

For calls received by the communications center via 9-1-1, the communications officers will take the call in accordance with normal Director Emergency Management (DEM) procedures. After the call is received, the communications center will advise field communications of the location, nature, and priority of the incident. **After field communications acknowledges receipt of the call, the communications center will cancel the call for computer-aided design (CAD) purposes.** Field communications will then dispatch the closest available standby unit to respond to the incident. If a transport unit is required, field communications will then advise the communications center of an evacuation point for the system ambulance to respond to.

**NO STANDBY UNITS ON SCENE ARE TO CONTACT
THE COMMUNICATIONS CENTER DIRECTLY EXCEPT IN CASE OF EMERGENCY.**

**ALL RESPONDING TEMS TRANSPORT UNITS WILL SWITCH TO EMS-3
AFTER DISPATCH AND BE HANDED OFF TO FIELD COMMUNICATIONS FOR
THE DURATION OF THE INCIDENT.**

Hospital Assignment Guidelines:

On the morning prior to race start, field communications will poll area facilities for their capabilities and the number of patients they can accept for each triage status. Field communications will assign transport units to facilities to evenly distribute patient load.

Patients transported from the north side of Martin Luther King Avenue/Franklin Street will be assigned to either:

- Medical Center Hospital;
- Oakwood Hospital; or
- Henry Ford Medical Center.

Patients transported from the south side of Martin Luther King Avenue/Franklin Street will be assigned to either:

- St. Mary's Medical Center;
- Providence Medical Center; or
- Annapolis Hospital.

Hospital assignments can be altered based on specialty resource needs. Field communications will document the destination of any participants transported.

MCI Response

In the event of an MCI, triage, treatment, and transportation will be handled in accordance with the County MCI plan, as well as local policy and protocol. Unified Command (UC) will expand the ICS structure as necessary, and establish triage and treatment areas for use by the operations section. The communications center will also dedicate an Emergency Communications Officer to the operation.

Medic Center must be immediately notified of the declaration of an MCI by phone at 313-123-4567.

MEDEVACs

If, due to patient condition, working MCI, or other contingency, a MEDEVAC is required, the following landing zones have been identified for MEDEVAC operations.

- Medical center helipad
  - Lat: 12°34'56" Lon: 67°89'10"
- Public soccer field
  - Lat: 12°34'56" Lon: 67°89'10"
- Baseball diamond
  - Lat: 12°34'56" Lon: 67°89'10"

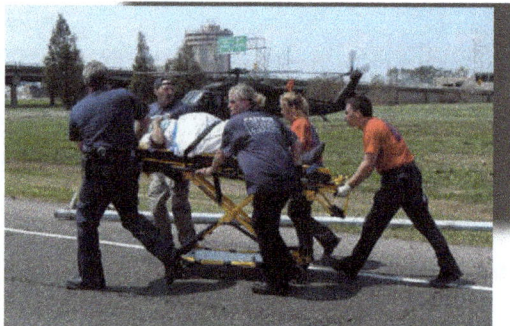

Emergency workers begin moving a rescued evacuee to the medical triage area after being rescued by a medevac helicopter.

Other Contingencies

Other contingencies encountered during the event are to be handled in accordance with TEMS standard operating procedures and policies and at the direction of UC.

Annex II: Sample Mass Gathering Event Planning Tools

Sample After Action Report

Townville Marathon
September 29, 2011

Table of Contents

Executive Summary 122
Event Details 122
Background 122
Medical Support 122
Command and Control 122
Incident and Patient Statistics 123
    Overall Patient Statistics 123
    Patient Breakdown by Complaint 123
    Patient Breakdown by Event 123
Response Missions and Outcomes.. 124
Conclusions... 126
Attachments.. 127

Executive Summary

The 30th running of the Townville Marathon occurred on September 29, 2011. Every year, this event poses unique challenges for the Townville EMS (TEMS) system, ranging from logistics to status planning to communications. This year, our personnel applied new ideas in the planning and execution of our response to this event, with mainly positive results.

The event consisted of separate races, the Shriners 8k run and the Townville Marathon. The event had a record attendance of 11,742 participants, with another 30,000 spectators estimated to have attended. A total of 96 people requested medical assistance, with 7 patients requiring transport.

Our response to the event highlighted improvements in command, control, and communications (C3) for special events. The use of a custom C3 application and special radio interoperability equipment enhanced situational awareness for both command elements and line personnel. Field data collection has provided a means for enhanced after-action analysis and reporting.

No response, however, is perfect. Several areas requiring improvement were identified, some within our control and some not. These areas include increasing the involvement of event organizers in preplanning and enhancing communications with other responding agencies, such as the Police Department.

Event Details

Background

The 2011 Townville Marathon drew a higher participant and spectator base due, in part, to the 30th anniversary celebrations going on at various parts of the course. There were approximately five "party stops" along the course, providing live music, food, and beverages to spectators, along with large "party areas" at the start and finish lines.

Specific information on the event is as follows:

Race Length: 26.2 miles

Registered Participants: 11,742

Spectators: 30,000 (estimated)

Weather at Start: Cloudy, 36 °F, with N winds at 16MPH.

Weather at Finish: Sunny, 50 °F, with N winds at 10MPH.

Medical Support

Medical support was provided by TEMS agency personnel and Wayne Ambulance personnel, as well as personnel from area hospitals. Four ALS ambulances, three ALS bike teams, and one ALS Echo Unit were present along the course, along with two fixed medical facilities provided by Henry Ford Medical Center.

All ambulances and bike teams were staffed to the Paramedic level and were sufficiently equipped to provide ALS care. The fixed medical facilities were staffed by a mix of physicians, registered nurses, athletic trainers, and medical students and were also equipped to provide high-level ALS care.

Command and Control

Command and Control was accomplished via a field command and communications center set up at the main medical facility. This facility included laptops with mobile data connectivity, radio interoperability equipment, maps, cellular phones, and radios.

Annex II: Sample Mass Gathering Event Planning Tools

Radio interoperability was achieved by using the Incident Commander's Radio Interface (ICRI), manufactured by Communications-Applied Technology (C-AT). The ICRI used was provided by C-AT as a demonstration unit, to evaluate its efficacy in our operational environment.

Command of the incident was functionally handled by Battalion Chief Chester Arthur, with Captain James Polk present to provide senior-level operational guidance and to liaise with other responding agencies.

Incident and Patient Statistics

Overall Patient Statistics

# Patients by EMS	# Patients by Med Facility	# Patients Transported
17	79	7
Avg. Patient Age	# Male Patients	# Female Patients
34	42 (43.75%)	54 (56.25%)
Age Youngest Patient	Age Oldest Patient	Average EMS Response Time
8	60	4.8 Min

Patient Breakdown by Complaint

Abdominal Pain:	2	2.0%
Breathing Problem:	4	4.2%
Chest Pain:	4	4.2%
Heart Problem:	2	2.0%
Sick Person:	48	50.0%
Traumatic Injury:	27	28.1%
Unconscious/Syncope:	9	9.4%

Patient Breakdown by Event

Percentage of Participants Requiring Care	0.8%
Percentage of Patients Requiring Transport	7.3%
Number of Transports to Number of Attendees	1:5,963
Percentage of Daily Transports* from Event	6.8%
Percentage of System Transports During Event**	13.2%
Calls per Standby Unit	1.9

* Total system transports for 24-hour period.
** Event period from 0700 thru 1500 hours.

Response Missions and Outcomes

TEMS personnel had several missions for the planning and execution of our response to this event. The following missions were identified:

1. Create a solid operations plan for the event, addressing most likely risks.
2. Staff the event to a level that permits continued compliance with response time standards.
3. Minimize event impact on the overall Townville EMS system.
4. Establish an effective command, control, and communications infrastructure.
5. Provide exceptional clinical care to event participants.
6. Provide for the rapid evacuation of casualties requiring transport.

An analysis of each mission and its outcome follows, along with recommendations for improvement.

Mission 1: Create a solid operations plan for the event, addressing most likely risks.

General Outcome: Success.

Discussion: Approximately one month pre-event, Captain James Polk, Martin Buren, and Chester Arthur began the preplanning process for the event. An online project management application, known as Basecamp, was used with great success. The application allowed the planners, who all worked different shifts on different days, to collaborate effectively during the planning phase of the operation.

The plan was authored primarily by Chester Arthur, with input from Captain Polk and Sgt. Buren. The plan was designed to address most contingencies encountered during the response to past events, as well as ones not previously encountered or planned for. The plan addressed everything from the initial command structure, to a preplanned MCI response, to MEDEVAC landing zones.

Sports Group personnel stated they were unfamiliar with the ICS used during the event and wished to learn more about it.

Recommendations for Improvement: Provide training to senior-level personnel at Townville Sports Group in the ICS and how to function as part of a UC. Also, insist on more involvement on the part of the Sports Group in the planning phase of our operations.

Mission 2: Staff the event to a level that permits continued compliance with response time standards.

General Outcome: Success.

Discussion: Townville Sports Group requested and paid for a total of six units (three Ambulances and three Bike Teams) from the TEMS agency to provide EMS services during the event. The TEMS provided these resources, staffed to the ALS level. Augmenting these resources was an ALS ambulance provided by the Wayne Ambulance.

Staffing for this year's event appeared to be appropriate; standby units averaged 1.9 calls per unit, with an average response time of 4.8 minutes. There are, however, anecdotal reports that this year's patient volume was lighter than usual; some long-time staff report that volume was up to one half of what has been experienced in the past.

Recommendations for Improvement: Continue to collect patient volume data from future events to improve our planning capabilities.

Mission 3: Minimize event impact on the overall TEMS system.
General Outcome: Success.

Discussion: The impact on the TEMS system as a whole appeared to be moderate. The only resources required from the system were used to transport patients from the event; these transports accounted for more than 13 percent of all transports during the event period and almost 7 percent of total transports for the day.

Recommendations for Improvement: Increase system staffing during future events by 1 or 2 units.

Mission 4: Establish an effective command, control, and communications infrastructure.
General Outcome: Success.

Discussion: A C3 facility was established on site, with all event communications going through that facility. This facility was established at the main medical facility and included mobile data connectivity, radio interoperability equipment, maps, cellular telephones, and a variety of radio equipment.

C3 personnel's situational awareness was enhanced by a custom incident management application designed, coded, and deployed by Chester Arthur. This application tracked units, unit status, times, patient contacts, and logged events. This approach has proven effective during both past events and the Marathon. Because of its proven efficacy, further development of this application is warranted.

Radio interoperability was achieved by use of the ICRI, manufactured by C-AT. C-AT provided a demonstration unit for us to test and evaluate during this event, and it performed flawlessly. Using the ICRI, units from TEMS, Monroe, and Sports Group were able to communicate seamlessly.

One problem encountered from a C3 standpoint was communications between EMS Operations and Police Operations. Information had to be relayed through Captain Polk, resulting in delays in essential information getting to the appropriate resources.

Another problem encountered during the event involved Sports Group personnel not knowing how or where to request medical resources. Sports Group personnel were apparently given multiple phone numbers to call, often resulting in requests being delayed.

Radio communications and data connectivity were hampered by the location of the C3 facility. Because the facility was located inside a concrete parking structure, intermittent outages in radio and data communications were experienced. While inconvenient, it posed no significant problems in C3 activities.

Recommendations for Improvement: Support further development of an incident management application for use during emergencies and special events. Explore the acquisition of one or more ICRI units for special events and disaster preparedness. Ensure that EMS personnel are involved in the briefing of Sports Group personnel, so that appropriate contact information and procedures are relayed. Ensure that future C3 facilities are located in an area that minimizes radio and cellular interference.

Mission 5: Provide exceptional clinical care to event participants.
General Outcome: Success.

Discussion: Henry Ford Medical Center provided a significant number of medical providers and equipment for the establishment of onsite treatment facilities. These facilities were staffed with high-level providers, including Physicians and Nurse Practitioners. Sufficient bed space was available in these facilities, with no more than 50 percent of bed space being occupied at one time.

One problem encountered during the event was a lack of some durable medical equipment, such as cardiac monitors. Some equipment had to be taken from the standby units, which would have prevented the onsite medical staff from using that equipment if the standby unit needed to transport a patient.

Recommendations for Improvement: Continue to work with Henry Ford Medical Center personnel to further enhance onsite treatment facilities. Ensure that sufficient durable equipment is available for future events.

Mission 6: Provide for the rapid evacuation of casualties requiring transport.
General Outcome: Success.

Discussion: The location and configuration of the medical sites, along with on-the-fly coordination with Police units allowed for easy ingress and egress of transporting units. While not used, preplanned landing zones for MEDEVAC assets were identified and forwarded to area aeromedical units. No significant delays in patient transportation were noted.

Recommendations for Improvement: Continue to work closely with local Police and aeromedical resources to ensure timely transport of casualties from the event.

Conclusions

While opportunities for improvement are apparent, the operation can be considered an overall success. TEMS personnel should continue to research, develop, and deploy new methods and technologies to enhance our response to not only future Marathons, but to any large-scale special event or emergency.

Annex II: Sample Mass Gathering Event Planning Tools

Attachments—Sample Incident Action Plan

Townville Marathon
September 29, 2011

INCIDENT OBJECTIVES (ICS FORM 202)

1. Incident Name: Townville Marathon	2. Operational Period:	Date From: 9/29/11 Time From: 0600	Date To: 9/29/11 Time To: 1600

3. Objective(s):

Reduce the risk of injuries or illnesses occurring as a result of the upcoming marathon.

Provide clear information to attendees and participants on how to obtain assistance if they encounter an illness or injury.

Establish methods for attendees and event workers to communicate with onscene medical personnel.

Respond to requests for assistance in a safe and appropriate manner.

4. Operational Period Command Emphasis:

Encourage each other to drink plenty of fluids, stay in the shade when possible, use all available personal protective equipment. Be extremely cautious of pedestrians when operating motor vehicles in or around crowds. Absolutely no backing without a spotter while on the course.

General Situational Awareness

Weather Update: Winds 5 mph WSW, humidity 80-85%, temperature 90 °F, sunny, 20% chance of precipitation. No storms predicted.

5. Site Safety Plan Required? Yes ❏ No X

  Approved Site Safety Plan(s) Located at:

6. Incident Action Plan (the items checked below are included in this Incident Action Plan):

X ICS 203	X ICS 207	Other Attachments:
X ICS 204	❏ ICS 208	❏ _____
X ICS 205	❏ Map/Chart	❏ _____
❏ ICS 205A	❏ Weather Forecast/Tides/Currents	❏ _____
X ICS 206		❏ _____

7. Prepared by: Name: William Taft   Position/Title: Planning Section Chief   Signature:

8. Approved by Incident Commander: Name: Zachary Taylor Signature:_____

ICS 202	IAP Page __1__	Date/Time: 7/29/11 0800

ORGANIZATION ASSIGNMENT LIST (ICS FORM 203)

1. Incident Name: Townville Marathon		2. Operational Period:	Date From: 9/29/11 Time From: 0600		Date To: 9/29/11 Time To: 1600
3. Incident Commander(s) and Command Staff:			**7. Operations Section:**		
IC/UCs	Wayne Harding		Chief	James Polk	
			Deputy		
Deputy			Staging Area		
Safety Officer	James Buchanan		**Group**	EMS	
Public Info. Officer	Benjamin Harrison		Group Supervisor	Sgt. Martin Buren	
Liaison Officer	Franklin Pierce		Deputy		
4. Agency/Organization Representatives:			Division/Group	Townville EMS	
Agency/Organization	Name		Division/Group	Monroe EMS	
Townville EMS Agency	James Polk		Division/Group	Wayne EMS	
Monroe EMS	William McKinley		Division/Group	TEMS Bike Team	
Wayne EMS	Millard Fillmore		Division/Group	TFD Bike Team	
			Group	Onsite Medical	
			Group Supervisor	Dr. Grant	
			Deputy		
5. Planning Section:			Division/Group	Nursing Staff	
Chief	Bill Taft		Division/Group	Sports Trainers	
Deputy			Division/Group	Ancillary Staff	
Resources Unit			Division/Group		
Situation Unit			Division/Group		
Documentation Unit			**Group**		
Demobilization Unit			Group Supervisor		
Technical Specialists			Deputy		
			Division/Group		
			Division/Group		
6. Logistics Section:			Division/Group		
Chief			Division/Group		
Deputy			**Air Operations Branch**		
Support Branch			Air Ops Branch Dir.		
Director					
Supply Unit					
Facilities Unit			**8. Finance/Administration Section:**		
Ground Support Unit			Chief		
Service Branch			Deputy		
Director			Time Unit		
Communications Unit			Procurement Unit		
Medical Unit			Comp/Claims Unit		
Food Unit			Cost Unit		

9. Prepared by: Name: William Taft   Position/Title: Planning Section Chief   Signature: _____

ICS 203   IAP Page __2__   Date/Time: 7/29/11 0800

Annex II: Sample Mass Gathering Event Planning Tools

ASSIGNMENT LIST (ICS FORM 204)

1. Incident Name: Townville Marathon	2. Operational Period: Date From: 9/29/11 Date To: 9/29/11 Time From: 0600 Time To: 1600		3. Branch: Division: Group: EMS Staging Area:
4. Operations Personnel:	Name	Contact Number(s)	
Operations Section Chief:	James Polk	xxx-xxx-xxxx	
Branch Director:		xxx-xxx-xxxx	
Division/Group Supervisor:	Martin Buren		

5. Resources Assigned:				
Resource Identifier	Leader	# of Persons	Contact (e.g., phone, pager, radio frequency, etc.)	Reporting Location, Special Equipment and Supplies, Remarks, Notes, Information
TEMS Amb 1	JH	2	TEMS_EMS3	TEMS HQ/0600
TEMS Amb 2	TY	2	TEMS_EMS3	TEMS HQ/0600
Wayne Amb	RF	3	TEMS_EMS3	TEMS HQ/0600
Monroe Amb	DJ	2	TEMS_EMS3	TEMS HQ/0600
TEMS Bike Team 1	IP	2	TEMS_EMS3	TEMS HQ/0600
TEMS Bike Team 2	YM	2	TEMS_EMS3	TEMS HQ/0600
TFD Bike Team 3	HN	2	TEMS_EMS3	TEMS HQ/0600

6. Work Assignments:

Bike team leaders must ensure all equipment is checked and loaded into assigned ambulance no later than 0615

7. Special Instructions:

Use extreme caution near race course; participants may not notice emergency vehicles due to loud background noise and visual distractions.

8. Communications (radio and/or phone contact numbers needed for this assignment):
Name/Function   Primary Contact: indicate cell, pager, or radio (frequency/system/channel)

_____ / _____   _____

_____ / _____   _____

_____ / _____   _____

_____ / _____   _____

9. Prepared by: Name: William Taft   Position/Title: Planning Sec Chief   Signature: _____

ICS 204	IAP Page __3__	Date/Time: 7/29/11 0800

ASSIGNMENT LIST (ICS FORM 204)

1. Incident Name: Townville Marathon	2. Operational Period: Date From: 9/29/11 Date To: 9/29/11 Time From: 0600 Time To: 1400	3. Branch: Division: 1 Group: On-Site Medical Staging Area: Parking Structure

4. Operations Personnel:

	Name	Contact Number(s)
Operations Section Chief:	James Polk	xxx-xxx-xxxx
Branch Director:		xxx-xxx-xxxx
Division/Group Supervisor:	Dr. Grant	xxx-xxx-xxx

5. Resources Assigned:

Resource Identifier	Leader	# of Persons	Contact (e.g., phone, pager, radio frequency, etc.)	Reporting Location, Special Equipment and Supplies, Remarks, Notes, Information
Medical Tent	Dr. Carter	8	TEMS_EMS2	TEMS HQ / 0600
Mobile Medical	Dr. Johnson	2	TEMS_EMS2	TEMS HQ / 0600

6. Work Assignments:

Medical team leaders must ensure all equipment is checked and loaded into assigned ambulance no later than 0615

7. Special Instructions:

Use care setting up medical area to avoid trip and electrical hazards. Store oxygen tanks in a safe location.
Use extreme caution near race course, participants may not notice emergency vehicles due to loud background noise and visual distractions.

8. Communications (radio and/or phone contact numbers needed for this assignment):

Name/Function   Primary Contact: indicate cell, pager, or radio (frequency/system/channel)

_____ / _____   _____
_____ / _____   _____
_____ / _____   _____
_____ / _____   _____

9. Prepared by: Name: William Taft   Position/Title: Planning Sec Chief   Signature: _____

ICS 204   IAP Page __3A__   Date/Time: 7/29/11 0800   _____

Annex II: Sample Mass Gathering Event Planning Tools

INCIDENT RADIO COMMUNICATIONS PLAN (ICS FORM 205)

1. Incident Name: Townville Marathon

2. Date/Time Prepared:
Date: 7/29/11
Time: 0800

3. Operational Period:
Date Form: 9/29/11   Date To: 9/29/11
Time Form: 0600   Time To: 1600

4. Basic Radio Channel Use:

Zone Grp.	Ch #	Function	Channel Name/Trunked Radio System Talkgroup	Assignment	RX Freq N or W	RX Tone/NAC	TX Freq N or W	TX Tone/NAC	Mode (A, D, or M)	Remarks
A	3	Command	TEMS_EMS3	Branch 1, Group A		N/A			A	
A	1	Support	TAC_1	Branch 1, Group A		N/A			M	
N/A	9	MCI Comms	MED_9	Command Only					A	

5. Special Instructions:
Hospital assignments for transport units will occur through operations.

6. Prepared by (Communications Unit Leader): Name: James Polk   Signature: _____   Date/Time: 7/29/11 0800

ICS 205   IAP Page ___4___

MEDICAL PLAN (ICS FORM 206)

1. Incident Name: Townville Marathon	2. Operational Period:	Date From: 9/29/11	Date To: 9/29/11
		Time From: 0600	Time To: 1600

3. Medical Aid Stations:

Name	Location	Contact Number(s)/Frequency	Paramedics on Site?
Primary Treatment	20th and Main	xxx-xxx-xxxx	❏ Yes X No
Secondary Treatment		xxx-xxx-xxxx	❏ Yes X No
			❏ Yes ❏ No
			❏ Yes ❏ No

4. Transportation (indicate air or ground):

Ambulance Service	Location	Contact Number(s)/Frequency	Level of Service
Townville EMS	123 Main St., Townville, MI	xxx-xxxx	X ALS ❏ BLS
Monroe EMS	45 Michigan Ave., Warren, MI	xxx-xxxx	X ALS ❏ BLS
Wayne EMS	23900 Ford Rd., Dearborn, MI	xxx-xxxx	X ALS ❏ BLS
			❏ ALS ❏ BLS

5. Hospitals:

Hospital Name	Address, Latitude and Longitude if Helipad	Contact Number(s)/ Frequency	Travel Time Air	Travel Time Ground	Trauma Center	Burn Center	Helipad
Medical Center Hospital			20m	15m	X Yes Level: __I__	X Yes ❏ No	X Yes ❏ No
Oakwood Hospital			20m	25m	❏ Yes Level: _____	❏ Yes X No	X Yes ❏ No
Henry Ford Medical Center			25m	30m	X Yes Level: __I__	❏ Yes X No	X Yes ❏ No
					❏ Yes Level: _____	❏ Yes ❏ No	❏ Yes ❏ No
					❏ Yes Level: _____	❏ Yes ❏ No	❏ Yes ❏ No

6. Special Medical Emergency Procedures:
Ambulances are not permitted to transport patients from a scene to onsite Primary Treatment area. If transported, these patients must be transported to a full-service hospital.

❏ Check box if aviation assets are utilized for rescue. If assets are used, coordinate with Air Operations.

7. Prepared by (Medical Unit Leader): Name: Dr. Grant   Signature: _____

8. Approved by (Safety Officer): Name: Grover Cleveland   Signature: _____

ICS 206   IAP Page ___5___   Date/Time: 7/29/11 0800

Annex II: Sample Mass Gathering Event Planning Tools

INCIDENT ORGANIZATION CHART (ICS FORM 207)

1. Incident Name: Townville Marathon

2. Operational Period: Date From: 9/29/11　Date To: 9/29/11　Time From: 06:00　Time To: 14:00

3. Organization Chart

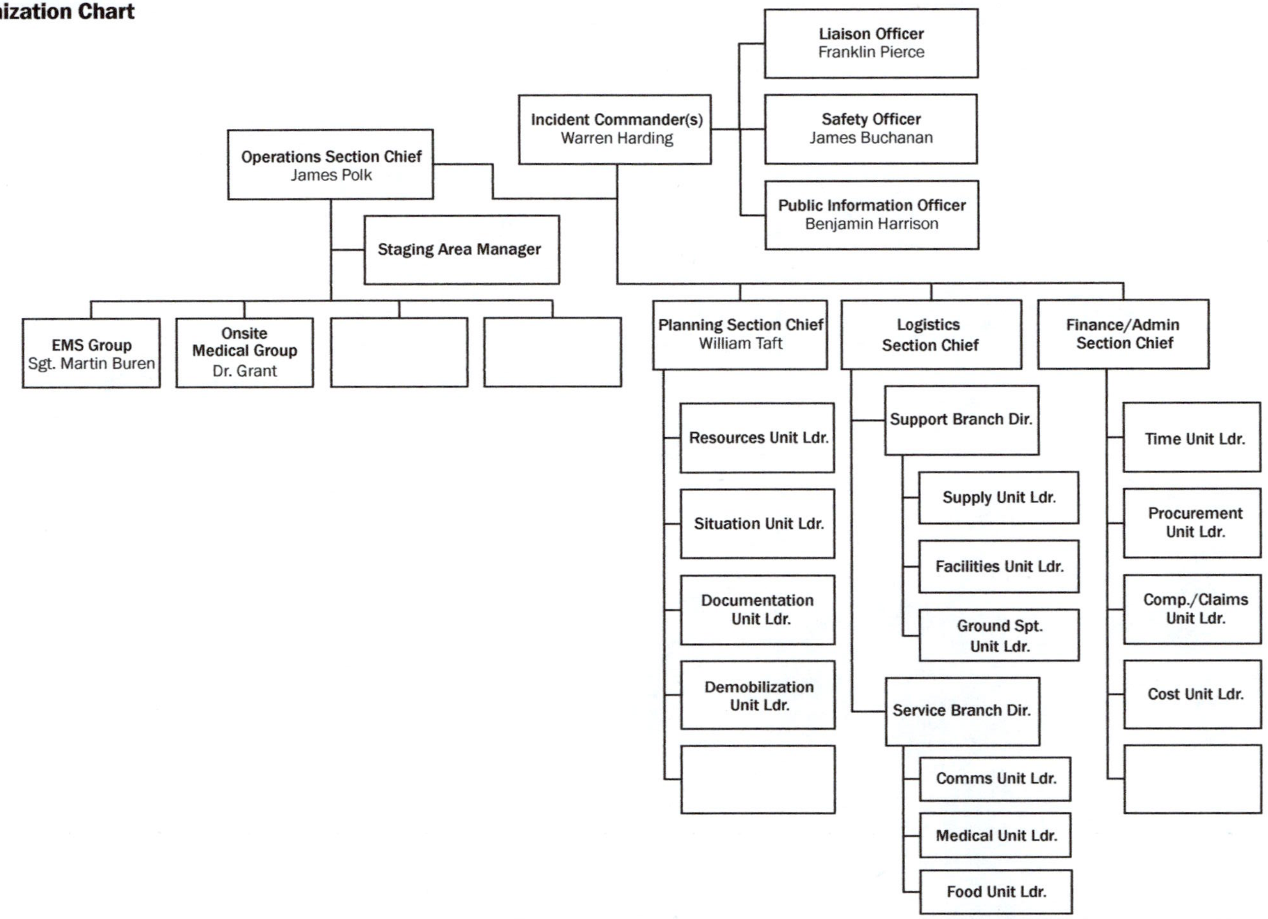

- **Incident Commander(s)** — Warren Harding
  - Liaison Officer — Franklin Pierce
  - Safety Officer — James Buchanan
  - Public Information Officer — Benjamin Harrison
  - **Operations Section Chief** — James Polk
    - Staging Area Manager
    - Onsite Medical Group — Dr. Grant
    - EMS Group — Sgt. Martin Buren
  - **Planning Section Chief** — William Taft
    - Resources Unit Ldr.
    - Situation Unit Ldr.
    - Documentation Unit Ldr.
    - Demobilization Unit Ldr.
  - **Logistics Section Chief**
    - Support Branch Dir.
      - Supply Unit Ldr.
      - Facilities Unit Ldr.
      - Ground Spt. Unit Ldr.
    - Service Branch Dir.
      - Comms Unit Ldr.
      - Medical Unit Ldr.
      - Food Unit Ldr.
  - **Finance/Admin Section Chief**
    - Time Unit Ldr.
    - Procurement Unit Ldr.
    - Comp./Claims Unit Ldr.
    - Cost Unit Ldr.

4. Prepared by: Name: William Taft　**Position/Title:** Planning　**Signature:** _____　**Date/Time:** 7/29/11 0800

ICS 207　IAP Page __6__

This page was intentionally left blank.

ANNEX III: Emergency Management Assistance Compact

Description

Emergency Management Assistance Compact (EMAC) is a national interstate mutual aid agreement that enables States to share resources during times of disaster. Since the 104th Congress ratified the compact, EMAC has grown to become the Nation's system for providing mutual aid through operational procedures and protocols that have been validated through experience. EMAC is administered by the National Emergency Management Association (NEMA).

EMAC Fast Facts

- EMAC acts as a complement to the Federal disaster response system.
- EMAC can be used either in lieu of Federal assistance or in conjunction with Federal assistance.
- EMAC ensures appropriate use of resources within member States.
- EMAC has been adopted by all 50 States, the District of Columbia, the U.S. Virgin Islands, and Puerto Rico.
- EMAC has been ratified by Congress (PL-104-321).

Process for EMS Agency Participation

The process for participation in EMAC is governed by the specific legislation in each State that authorized entry of the State into the compact. In general terms, an agency must enter into a contract with the agency's State. The contract should contain specific elements that improve coordination of resources including the process for deployment, communications during the deployment, worker safety, demobilization procedures, and reimbursement. Obtaining competent legal advice from an attorney familiar with State level contracting, particularly contracting that involves emergency operations is important.

The contract must be in line with State legislation. The contract should be executed prior to deployment to avoid any delay in deploying while the contracting process takes place. Components of a State Agency contract are included in the following checklist.

EMAC CONTRACTING CHECKLIST	
COMPLETE	**ELEMENT**
	Name of Agency
	Name of State Agency
	Purpose and Goal
	Authority in State Law
	Points of Contact
	Definitions
	Resource Typing
	Credentialing
	Agency Licensure and/or Certification
	Medical Direction and Protocols
	Mobilization Notification and Authority
PERFORMANCE STANDARDS	
COMPLETE	**ELEMENT**
	Mobilization Time
	Deployment Duration
	Staffing Standards Based on Resource Typing
	Equipment
	Personal Protective Equipment (PPE)
	Training Requirements
	Communications Requirements
	Physical/Medical Requirements and Immunizations
REIMBURSEMENT	
COMPLETE	**ELEMENT**
	Language Specifying Reimbursement is "Portal to Portal"
	Labor (Including Overtime)
	Labor Replacement Costs (Backfill)
	Travel and Lodging
	Fuel
	Supplies
	Food
	Equipment Rental
	Repairs
	Consider Using Mission Packaging Approach that Establishes an All-Inclusive Hourly/Daily Rate Per Unit for Known Expenses Based on Resource Type
OTHER PROVISIONS	
COMPLETE	**ELEMENT**
	Dispute Resolution
	Immunity, Limited Liability, and Hold Harmless
	Death Benefits
	Workers' Compensation
	Length of Deployment
	Replacement
	Demobilization Authority and Responsibilities
	Documentation Requirements

EMAC Operational Considerations

Credentialing

EMAC uses the legislative framework and the compact itself to provide a form of temporary recognition for licensees from one State rendering requested aid in another State. The specific language used in Article V of the Articles of Agreement is in part:

> Whenever any person holds a license, certificate, or other permit issued by any State party to the compact evidencing the meeting of qualifications for professional, mechanical, or other skills, and when such assistance is requested by the receiving party State, such person shall be deemed licensed, certified, or permitted by the State requesting assistance to render aid involving such skill to meet a declared emergency or disaster, subject to such limitations and conditions as the governor of the requesting State may prescribe by executive order or otherwise.

Deployment Process

As an appointed EMAC Authorized Representative, a State's highest ranking emergency management officer (most often a Director or Chief of Emergency Management) is empowered to request assistance under EMAC on behalf of the State. The process, once the authorized representative makes a request under EMAC, is outlined below.

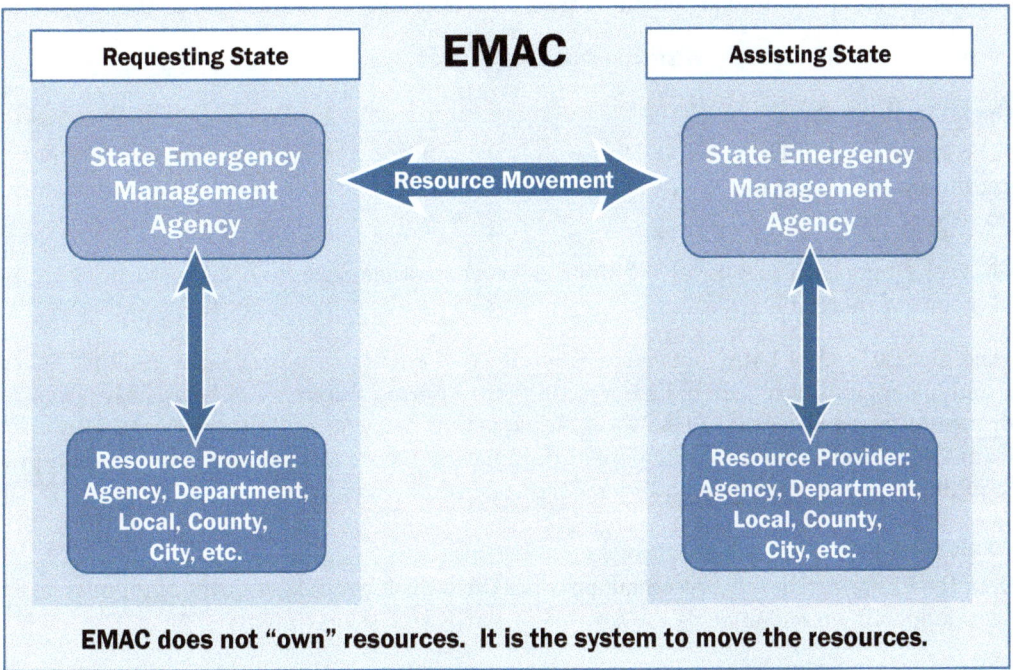

Authorized Representative confirms declaration of emergency by the Governor.

- State assesses needs for resources.
- State determines best source of resources (EMAC, Federal, private sector).
- Requests for resources may occur by one or all of the following methodologies:
  - Direct contact with a State that has a known needed resource;
  - EMAC Emergency Operations System (EOS); and

- States may request broadcast by region (FEMA regions):
    - May request up to 3 FEMA regions,
    - Broadcast to an individual State,
    - Directed to an individual EMAC Authorized Representative within a State,
    - Directed to an EMAC Designated Contact within a State.
- The EMAC REQ-A Form is completed by the EMAC Authorized Representatives in both the Requesting State and the Assisting State.
- Resources are mobilized from the Assisting State to the Requesting State.
- Resources check in at State staging areas. Deployment locations and missions are confirmed.
- Resources complete mission–relaying any issues back to their home State emergency management agency.
- Resources are demobilized.
- Assisting States complete reimbursement request, and after internal audit, send to the Requesting State.
- Requesting State reimburses the Assisting State.

EMAC Operational Levels

Level 3–The lowest level of EMAC activation involves the activation of the Assisting State, the National Coordination Group (NCG), and the NEMA EMAC Coordinator. The Assisting State is using their internal State A-Team to request resources.

Level 2–A level 2 operation may involve a single-State or multiple States and deployment of an A-Team is requested by one or more affected States.

Level 1–The highest level of EMAC activation is in effect whenever a single-State or multiple States within single or multiple regions have suffered a major disaster requiring resources. A-Teams have been requested by one or more affected States and DHS/FEMA Headquarters has requested that an EMAC National Coordinating Team (NCT) and/or an EMAC Regional Coordinating Team (RCT) be deployed to appropriate locations to coordinate resource needs with Federal and State counterparts.

Reimbursement

Article IX of the EMAC Articles of Agreement provides the basis for reimbursement of services provided between States following an activation of the agreement. Article IX states in part:

> *Any party State rendering aid in another State pursuant to this compact shall be reimbursed by the party State receiving such aid for any loss or damage to or expense incurred in the operation of any equipment and the provision of any service in answering a request for aid and for the costs incurred in connection with such requests; provided, that any aiding party State may assume in whole or in part such loss, damage, expense, or other cost, or may loan such equipment or donate such services to the receiving party State without charge or cost; and provided further, that any two or more party States may enter into supplementary agreements establishing a different allocation of costs among those States.*

Recordkeeping and other requirements to document expenses at the agency level vary from State to State. This underscores the necessity of having clear language in the contract between the EMS agency and the State so that terms and requirements for reimbursement are clear. Of particular note is the requirement for original receipts to validate claimed expenses, and a clear timeline for reimbursement between the State and the EMS agency.

Liability Protections

EMAC has standard language contained in Article VI of the Articles of Agreement that describes the limits on liability agreed to by each member State. In addition, each State may have liability limitations built into the EMAC authorizing legislation, or contained within the State's general emergency management legislation. In addition to the language in Article VI and any legislative protections, EMS agencies should include specific indemnity and liability protection language in their individual contract with the State. The liability language from Article VI states in part:

> *Officers or employees of a party State rendering aid in another State pursuant to this compact shall be considered agents of the requesting State for tort liability and immunity purposes; and no party State or its officers or employees rendering aid in another State pursuant to this compact shall be liable on account of any act or omission in good faith on the part of such forces while so engaged or on account of the maintenance or use of any equipment or supplies in connection therewith. Good faith in this article shall not include willful misconduct, gross negligence, or recklessness.*

EMAC Resources

- GAO Report to the Committee on Homeland Security and Governmental Affairs, U.S. Senate. *Emergency Management Assistance Compact: Enhancing EMAC's Collaborative and Administrative Capacity Should Improve National Disaster Response.* June 2007.

- Emergency Management Assistance Compact. *2005 Hurricane Season Response After Action Report.* Titan-L3. September 2006.

This page was intentionally left blank.

ANNEX IV: FEMA National Ambulance Contract

Description

Following the catastrophic 2005 hurricane season, Federal Emergency Management Agency (FEMA) sought to implement a plan to establish a comprehensive Emergency Medical Services (EMS) response to federally declared disasters. The government solicited proposals and on August 1, 2007, FEMA named American Medical Response (AMR) as the provider recipient of this contract, which provides a full array of ground ambulance, air ambulance, and paratransit services to supplement the Federal and military response to a disaster, act of terrorism, or other public health emergency. This national contract covers the 48 contiguous United States which are divided into 4 FEMA zones.

FEMA National Ambulance Contract Fast Facts

- Contracted services provided in this agreement include:
    - patient triage, treatment, and transport;
    - hazard recognition;
    - symptom surveillance and reporting;
    - onscene medical standby;
    - redistribution of patients to increase hospital bed space;
    - provide immunizations;
    - staffing for shelters and hospital emergency departments;
    - set up mobile medical clinics;
    - tactical management functions; and
    - oversight and management of Federal EMS and paratransit resources.

Deployment Capabilities and Contract Requirements

- Maximum deployment for a single FEMA zone includes:
    - 300 ground ambulances;
    - 25 air ambulances; and
    - enough paratransit vehicles to transport 3,500 people.
- Combined four-zone maximum deployment includes:
    - 1,200 ground ambulances;
    - 100 air ambulances;
    - 14,000 paratransit seats; and
    - simultaneous response from multiple zones for catastrophic disasters may be required under this national contract.

List of Deployments
- FEMA Contract, South Louisiana, 2006.
- FEMA deployment Hurricane Dean, 2007.
- FEMA deployment Hurricane Gustav, 2008.
- FEMA deployment Hurricane Ike, 2008.
- FEMA deployment Presidential Inauguration, 2009.

Process for EMS Agency Participation

EMS agencies choosing to participate in the FEMA National Ambulance Contract must apply to become a subcontractor through the AMR Disaster Response Team. Agencies must be able to articulate which types of resources they can supply for deployment in addition to other terms and conditions. A checklist of preliminary information that the agency must have at the time of application is located below:

COMPLETE	FEMA NATIONAL AMBULANCE CONTRACT CHECKLIST
	ELEMENT
	Organization Name
	Complete Business Address
	Name and Title of the Primary Point of Contact
	Business, 24/7 Available, and Fax Phone Numbers
	Primary and Secondary Email Address
	States the Agency is Licensed
	Services Provided: ALS Ground Ambulance Service
	Services Provided: BLS Ground Ambulance
	Services Provided: Air Ambulance
	Services Provided: Paratransit
	Type of Service (Fire EMS, Government, Hospital Based, Private, PUM, Volunteer, Other)
	Determine Small Business Status (fewer than 500 employees)
	Does Agency Have an Equal Opportunity Employment Plan?
	Agency Registered as Woman Owned with the Small Business Administration?
	Agency Registered as Veteran Owned with the Small Business Administration?
	Agency Registered as Disabled Veteran Owned with the Small Business Administration?
	Agency Registered as HUB Zone Business with Small Business Administration?
	Agency Registered as Disadvantaged with Small Business Administration?
	National Accreditation Status and Name of Accrediting Body
	No officers or owners are prohibited from participating in any Federal program
	Agency can label internal resources according to FEMA type definitions

Jurisdiction

The National Response Framework (NRF) identifies FEMA as the Federal lead agency during an Incident of National Significance. Emergency Support Function-8 (ESF-8)—Public Health and Medical Services Annex— is the mechanism for coordinated Federal assistance to supplement State and local resources in response to the public health and medical care needs of potential or actual federally declared disasters and/or during a developing potential health and medical situation. The U.S. Department of Health and Human Services (DHHS) is the coordinating lead agency for the Federal Government on public health and medical services.

The FEMA national ambulance contract may be activated to provide supplemental EMS support when local and State resources are overwhelmed. FEMA and DHHS will coordinate the Federal EMS response. AMR will provide tactical command and oversight of resources deployed pursuant to the national contract. EMS providers are regulated by local or State agencies and may have restrictions when it comes to responding to out-of-area disasters. The EMS needs of local communities are primary and participation in the national ambulance contract is not intended to undermine those obligations.

Relationship between FEMA National Ambulance Contract and EMAC

States may have Emergency Management Assistance Compact (EMAC) agreements with EMS agencies. The FEMA National Ambulance Contract will not utilize assets that are committed under EMAC.

FEMA National Ambulance Contract Operational Considerations

Defining Resources and Job Titles

The FEMA Typed Resources Definitions, Emergency Medical Services Resources are used as a guideline for EMS responders. The applicable EMS job titles listed in FEMA's National Emergency Responder Credentialing document are used to determine the required and recommended training and certification. Both Advanced Life Support (ALS) and Basic Life Support (BLS) services are used. EMS personnel are required to maintain current credentials in their home State to practice at the required skill level.

Integration of the FEMA National Ambulance Contract with NIMS and the NRF

The National Incident Management System (NIMS) establishes standard incident management processes, protocols, and procedures to ensure that all responders work together more effectively. NIMS works hand-in-hand with the NRF. NIMS provides the template for the management of incidents, while the NRF provides the structure and mechanisms for national-level policy and incident management. The role of the FEMA National Ambulance Contract is to fulfill elements of ESF-8 within the NRF and integrate contracted assets into the overall incident management system employed to manage an event of national significance.

Standard of Care and Scope of Practice

For EMS deployments pursuant to the FEMA Contract, the National EMS Core Content will be used to define the domain of out-of-hospital care. The scope of practice for the FEMA Contract shall be the National EMS Scope of Practice Model.

FEMA National Ambulance Contract Resources

- AMR/FEMA/DHHS Paratransit Resource Utilization Guide.

This page was intentionally left blank.

ANNEX V: Intrastate Mutual Aid System

Description

This Intrastate Mutual Aid System (IMAS) is provided only as an example of how mutual aid across State lines is addressed in one specific instance. Each State is unique and this example may not be applicable to all jurisdictions.

Under the IMAS, member jurisdictions may request assistance from other member jurisdictions to prevent, mitigate, respond to, or recover from an emergency or disaster; or in concert with drills or exercises. Any resource (personnel, assets, and equipment) of a member jurisdiction may be made available to another member jurisdiction.

The goal of a national fire service mutual aid system is to create a venue in each of the 50 States that would ensure a comprehensive, coordinated response to any incident within, or immediately adjacent to, its borders. Creating and implementing such a response system, with an understanding of resources and capabilities, paves the way for a more integrated and efficient response in the event of a national disaster. Specifically, it ensures that the local fire service brings its exceptional skills, unique knowledge, and tactical resources to the table to support national strategies such as National Incident Management System (NIMS) and State-based efforts, such as Emergency Management Assistance Compact (EMAC). Further, its goal is:

- to formalize IMAS concepts into detailed, comprehensive and exercised mutual aid systems;
- provide an efficient and coordinated response in an all-hazards environment;
- prepare for responding to large-scale or concurrent events; and
- provide assistance in addressing budget shortfalls and initiating concepts central to interoperability.

Pursuant to the Intrastate Mutual Aid Act, IMAS is composed of and may be described as:

- guidelines and procedures for implementing mutual aid across State boundaries;
- actions taken in requesting aid for an emergency or disaster;
- actions taken in responding to a request for aid; and
- the committee and actions taken by the committee.

Funding

The IMAS program is funded by a $700,000 Cooperative Agreement from the National Integration Center within the Department of Homeland Security. The performance period is from March 1 to February 28 annually.

Process for Participation

Pursuant to the Intrastate Mutual Aid Act, every political subdivision of the State is automatically part of the IMAS. Participation in the system does not preclude member jurisdictions from entering into other agreements with other political subdivisions or Indian nations to the extent provided by law. Participation does not supersede nor affect any other agreement to which a political subdivision is a party or may become a party.

Participation becomes official upon receipt of a copy of the resolution by the authority responsible for the execution of the agreement (most often the State Office of Emergency Management). Member jurisdictions may elect to withdraw from or not participate in the system, but only by adopting a resolution or ordinance declaring these intentions. Withdrawal becomes official upon receipt of a copy of the resolution or ordinance by the State executing authority.

Steps for Participation and State Plan Development

- Plan Development (approximately 4 months).
  - plan created including Functional Components with buy-in from identified stakeholders in the State;
  - regional Coordinators identified by State;
  - appendices created; and
  - support from technical experts and International Association of Fire Chiefs (IAFC) staff.
- Marketing and Training (approximately 6–9 months).
  - field guide development; and
  - training and scripted tabletop exercise.
- Full-Scale Tabletop Exercise (approximately 12–14 months).
  - field guides (following plan development);
  - template review;
  - quick reference guide for Incident Commanders (ICs); and
  - useful grass roots marketing and training tool.

Lessons Learned from Successful Implementation of IMAS

- Importance of having emergency management within the IMAS State program (State and Local).
- Marketing of plan to all stakeholders.
- Clearly defined roles and responsibilities.
- Clearly defined reporting structure.
- Communications plan.
- Efficient operations between Emergency Support Functions (ESFs).
- Succession planning.
- Use of standardized tracking system(s).

Note Regarding Self-Deployment

The IMAS provides no immunity, rights, or privileges to individuals who respond to an emergency who are not requested and authorized to respond by member jurisdictions, in accordance with the Act.

Automatic Mutual Aid: Mutual Aid Box Alarm System (MABAS)

MABAS is an intrastate and interstate system used to provide automatic mutual aid across both the State of Illinois and the signed jurisdictions in the neighboring States of Indiana, Wisconsin, Missouri, and Iowa. During both day-to-day operations and during disasters, MABAS uses a system of protocols to initiate response of mutual aid assets in response to conditional criteria within the requesting jurisdiction.

MABAS has a response capability that includes almost 1,500 member fire departments and other agencies organized into 63 response divisions and 79 response units (engines, ladder trucks, ambulances, heavy and light rescue squads, water tankers, hazardous materials teams, underwater rescue and recovery teams, trench, building collapse, technical rescue teams, and certified fire investigators) that are resource typed and available upon request (Box Alarm Level I, Box Alarm Level II, Level III, task force, ambulance task force, etc.) via MABAS dispatch. Initial response is within the MABAS member response division, but additional resources can be obtained through neighboring divisions as well as through the Illinois Emergency Operations Plan. Resources through the Illinois Emergency Operations Plan require a disaster declaration while other day-to-day surge issues, such as mass gatherings or a mass casualty incident that does not reach the threshold where State involvement would be necessary, automatically occur within and across divisions through predetermined response protocols. Joining MABAS requires signing the same contract as other member organizations and agreeing to certain safety practices, standards of operation, onscene terminology incident command, equipment staffing, and conducting operations on common communications channels.

Over 850 MABAS extra alarm incidents occur annually through MABAS divisions. The MABAS parent organization support is cooperative. In addition to these other roles, MABAS trains 42 strategically placed hazardous materials response teams and 41 technical rescue teams across the State. Team members agree to become part of the team for five years, and the parent organization agrees to pay for member training costs, backfill, and overtime costs.

IMAS Resources

Resource Name	Website
IMAS Website	www.iafc.org/Programs/content.cfm?ItemNumber=1176
Model Agreements	www.iafc.org/Programs/content.cfm?ItemNumber=1157&navItemNumber=573
MABAS	www.mabas-il.org/Pages/WelcomeToMABAS.aspx

This page was intentionally left blank.

ANNEX VI: National Disaster Medical System-Disaster Medical Assistance Teams

Description

The National Disaster Medical System (NDMS) is a federally coordinated system that augments the Nation's medical response capability. The overall purpose of the NDMS is to supplement an integrated national medical response capability for assisting State and local authorities in dealing with the medical impacts of major peacetime disasters and to provide support to the military and the Department of Veterans Affairs medical systems in caring for casualties evacuated back to the United States from overseas armed conventional conflicts.

The National Response Framework (NRF) uses the NDMS, as part of the Department of Health and Human Services, Office of Preparedness and Response, under Emergency Support Function-8 (ESF-8), Health and Medical Services, to support Federal agencies in the management and coordination of the Federal medical response to major emergencies and federally declared disasters. Its components include:

- Disaster Medical Assistance Teams (DMAT);
- Disaster Mortuary Operational Response Teams (DMORT);
- National Veterinary Response Team (NVRT); and
- National Medical Response Team (NMRT).

Disaster Medical Assistance Teams (DMAT)

Description

A DMAT is composed of professional and paraprofessional medical personnel (supported by a cadre of logistical and administrative staff) designed to provide emergency medical care during a disaster or other event. In mass casualty incidents (MCIs), their responsibilities include triaging patients, providing austere medical care, and preparing patients for evacuation. In other situations, DMATs may provide primary health care or augment overloaded health care staffs.

Organization

There are 55 DMATs organized by State. Each is staffed by local groups of health care providers and support personnel that receive funding from the Federal government and other sources such as States, counties, and private donors. Under the NRF, DMATs are defined according to their level of capability and experience.

The typical DMAT is composed of physicians, nurse practitioners, physician assistants, nurses, pharmacists, respiratory therapists, paramedics, emergency medical technicians (EMTs), and a variety of other health and logistical personnel. DMATs typically have 50–125 total members, from which the Team Leader chooses 35 to deploy on most missions. A typical deployment might be composed of the following roles and specialty positions:

- **9 Nonclinical Positions**
    - 2 DMAT Leaders;
    - 1 Safety Officer;
    - 1 Administrative/Finance Chief;
    - 1 Administrative Assistant;

- 1 Logistics Chief;
- 1 Equipment Specialist; and
- 2 Communications Officers.

- **21 Clinical Positions**
  - 3 Medical Officers;
  - 1 Pharmacist;
  - 1 Pharmacy Assistant;
  - 2 Supervisory Nurse Specialists;
  - 6 Staff Nurses;
  - 4 Nurse Practitioners or Physician Assistants; and
  - 4 Paramedics.

- **6 Other Positions**
  - 5 other positions, determined by DMAT; and
  - 1 Home Base Support Person (activated, not deployed).

Although a standard deployment consists of approximately 35 positions, each particular team may consist of more than three times that number to provide some redundancy for each job role on the DMAT in the event a key person is unavailable at the time of deployment. Each DMAT is composed of members with a variety of health or medical skills. Included among the ranks of a team are many support personnel such as communications, logistics, maintenance, and security. Many teams also maintain a Critical Incident Stress Management (CISM) subunit.

DMAT Levels and Capabilities

For any DMAT, capability is designated within the name of the team. For instance, the Michigan DMAT team headquartered at Selfridge Air National Guard base is designated MI-1 DMAT defining it as a Level 1 team.

Level-1 ready to deploy within 8 hours of notification and then remain self-sufficient for 72 hours with enough food, water, shelter, and medical supplies to treat about 250 patients per day.

Level-2 ready to deploy and replace a Level-1 team using and supplementing their equipment which is left on site.

Level-3 teams in various stages of development.

Employment Status and Protections

DMAT members are defined as "intermittent" Federal employees, and once activated by Federal order, their status changes to that of an active Federal employee and follows the General Schedule (GS) pay scale. Federally activated DMAT members are protected from tort liability while in operation and are also protected by the provisions of the Uniformed Services Employment and Reemployment Rights Act (USERRA), which affords the same protections extended to National Guard and active duty military personnel in that when they deploy, their full-time jobs are not placed in jeopardy.

Process for Participation

Individual providers may apply for a position on a DMAT team through the administrative contact for a DMAT organization or through the NDMS website. The three-phase application process is described below.

PHASE 1:

- Applicant completes application for Federal employment through systems established by the Office of Personnel Management.
- Applicant must fill out NDMS Member Information form.
- Applicant provides true copies of education degrees and licenses for medical positions.
- Applicant provides true copies of Federal Emergency Management Agency (FEMA) Certificates of Completion for IS-100.b, IS-200.b, IS-700 and IS-800.b.
- Applicant completes the Direct Deposit Form and attaches a voided check.
- Applicant mails (or scans) all completed forms to DMAT team administrative officer contact.

PHASE 2:

- Local DMAT team and Department of Health and Human Services (DHHS) approve items from Phase 1.
- Applicant is fingerprinted and completes the Personal Identity Verification (PIV) Form.
- Applicant will receive an email from psc.hhs.gov to complete Electronic Questionnaire for Investigations Processing (e-QIP), the automated system for processing Federal applicant suitability investigations.
  - Applicants have 5 days to respond.
  - Applicant must follow all instructions regarding computer settings to complete this online process.
  - Applicants that do not complete the e-QIP process within two attempts will be required to reapply to NDMS as a NEW Applicant.
  - Three (3) e-QIP Signatory Forms must be completed (titled in lower right hand corner of each form).
    - Document type CER
    - Document type REL
    - Document type MEL
- Applicant completes and signs DHHS Credit Release Form.
- Applicant completes and signs Declaration of Federal Employment (Option Form 306).

PHASE 3:

- DMAT team receives confirmation that applicant's background check has been approved.
- **E-Induction**: Applicant is notified by email to complete the Online Induction process.
- Applicant completes required employment paperwork including letter of appointment.
- Applicant receives appointment as a member of DMAT.

DMAT RESOURCES

- NDMS/OEP. *National Disaster Medical System.* www.ndms.dhhs.gov (Retrieved July 3, 2011).

This page was intentionally left blank.

ANNEX VII: References

References and Reading List

Ablah, E., Konda, K.S., Konda, K., Melbourne, M., Ingoglia, J.N., and Gebbie, K.M. "Emergency Preparedness Training and Response among Community Health Centers and Local Health Departments: Results from a Multi-State Survey." Journal of Community Health 35, No. 3 (2010): 285-293.

AMR/FEMA/DHHS Paratransit Resource Utilization Guide.

Andreatta, P.B., Maslowski, E., Petty, S., Shim, W., Marsh, M., Hall, T., Stern, S., and Frankel, J. "Virtual Reality Triage Training Provides a Viable Solution for Disaster-Preparedness." Academic Emergency Medicine: Official Journal Of The Society For Academic Emergency Medicine 17, No. 8 (2010): 870-876.

Ariely, G. "Learning to digest during fighting—Real time knowledge management," http://www.instituteforcounterterrorism.org/apage/7572.php.

Barnes, M.D., Hanson, C.L., Novilla, L.M., Meacham, A.T., McIntyre, E., and Erickson, B.C. "Analysis of Media Agenda Setting During and after Hurricane Katrina: Implications for Emergency Preparedness, Disaster Response, and Disaster Policy." American Journal of Public Health 98, No. 4 (2008): 604-610.

"Catastrophic Disasters: Enhanced Leadership, Capabilities, and Accountability Controls Will Improve the Effectiveness of the Nation's Preparedness, Response, and Recovery System: Gao-06-618." GAO Reports, (2006): 1.

"Catastrophic Disasters: Gao-08-22." GAO Reports, (2008): 1.

Center for Catastrophe Preparedness and Response NYU. "Emergency Medical Services: The Forgotten First Responder—A Report on the Critical Gaps in Organization and Deficits in Resources for America's Medical First Responders." New York: New York University, 2005.

Chatham Emergency Management Agency. *After Action Report: Imperial Sugar Dixie Crystal Plant*, April 2008.

Cherry, R.A., and Trainer, M. "The Current Crisis in Emergency Care and the Impact on Disaster Preparedness." BMC Emergency Medicine 8, (2008): 1-7.

Chhabra, V. "Connecting Care Competencies and Culture During Disasters." Journal of Emergencies, Trauma & Shock 2, No. 2 (2009): 95-98.

City of Hartford After Action Report. *Motor Vehicle/Bus Accident I84 Westbound*, January 2010.

CLEMIS. *OAKWIN User Manual*, October 2005.

Collier, R. "Demystifying Radiation Disaster Preparedness." CMAJ: Canadian Medical Association Journal = Journal De L'association Medicale Canadienne 183, No. 9 (2011): 1002-1003.

Courtney, B. "Five Legal Preparedness Challenges for Responding to Future Public Health Emergencies." Journal of Law, Medicine & Ethics 39 (2011): 60-64.

Czerwinski, T. *Coping with the Bounds: Speculations on Nonlinearity in Military Affairs* (Washington, DC: DoD Command and Control Research Program, 1997), pp. 8-9.

Daughtery, L.G., and Blome, W.W. "Planning to Plan: A Process to Involve Child Welfare Agencies in Disaster Preparedness Planning." Journal of Community Practice 17, No. 4 (2009): 483-501.

Davies, K. "Disaster Management. Disaster Preparedness and Response: More Than Major Incident Initiation." British Journal of Nursing (BJN) 14, No. 16 (2005): 868-871.

de Hoop, T., and Ruben, R. "Insuring against Earthquakes: Simulating the Cost-Effectiveness of Disaster Preparedness." Disasters 34, No. 2 (2010): 509-523.

DHS (U.S. Department of Homeland Security). 2004. *National Response Plan*. Department of Homeland Security, Washington, DC.

_____. 2008a. *National Response Framework*. Department of Homeland Security, Washington, DC. Accessed at http://www.fema.gov/pdf/emergency/nrf/nrf-core.pdf on July 30, 2010.

_____. 2008b. *Mass Care, Emergency Assistance, Housing, and Human Services*, ESF 6. Department of Homeland Security, Washington, DC. Accessed at http://www.fema.gov/pdf/emergency/nrf/nrf-esf-06.pdf on July 30, 2010.

Dietrich, D. (1997). *The Logic of Failure: Recognizing and Avoiding Error in Complex Situations*. Rita and Robert Kimber, Trans. Cambridge, Massachusetts: Perseus Books.

Duggan, S.P., Deeny, R.S., and Vitale, C.T. "Perceptions of Older People on Disaster Response and Preparedness." International Journal of Older People Nursing 5, No. 1 (2010): 71-76.

Edwards, J.C., Kang, J., and Silenas, R. "Promoting Regional Disaster Preparedness among Rural Hospitals." The Journal Of Rural Health: Official Journal Of The American Rural Health Association And The National Rural Health Care Association 24, No. 3 (2008): 321-325.

Emergency Management Assistance Compact. *2005 Hurricane Season Response After Action Report*. Titan-L3. September 2006.

Endsley, M.R. 1995. "Toward a Theory of Situation Awareness in Dynamic Systems." *The Journal of the Human Factors and Ergonomics Society* 31 (1): 32-64.

Federal Emergency Management Agency. "Developing and Sustaining an Effective MMRS Regional System Hampton Roads, Virginia," FEMA Smart Practices Spotlight, October 15, 2003 (accessed April 27, 2011).

_____. "ICS-300: Intermediate ICS for Expanding Incidents (EMI Course Number: G300)." Emergency Management Institute, 2011.

_____. "ICS All Hazards Core Competencies." Emergency Management Institute, 2011.

Fox, M.H., White, G.W., Rooney, C., and Rowland, J.L. "Disaster Preparedness and Response for Persons with Mobility Impairments." Journal of Disability Policy Studies 17, No. 4 (2007): 196-205.

GAO Report to the Committee on Homeland Security and Governmental Affairs, U.S. Senate. *Emergency Management Assistance Compact: Enhancing EMAC's Collaborative and Administrative Capacity Should Improve National Disaster Response*. June 2007.

GAO (U.S. Government Accountability Office). 2003. *Geographic Information Systems*. Government Accountability Office, Washington, DC.

_____. 2005. *Results-Oriented Government: Practices That Can Help and Sustain Collaboration Among Federal Agencies*. Government Accountability Office, Washington, DC.

_____. 2006. *Hurricane Katrina: Better Plans and Exercises Needed to Guide the Military's Response to Natural Disasters*. Government Accountability Office, Washington, DC.

Annex VII: References

_____. 2007a. *Critical Infrastructure Protection: Progress Coordinating Government and Private Sector Efforts Varies by Sectors' Characteristics.* Government Accountability Office, Washington, DC.

_____. 2007b. *Homeland Security: Preliminary Information on Federal Actions to Address Challenges Faced by State and Local Information Fusion Centers.* Government Accountability Office, Washington, DC.

_____. 2007c. *Homeland Security: Observations on DHS and FEMA Efforts to Prepare for and Respond to Major and Catastrophic Disasters and Address Related Recommendations and Legislation.* Government Accountability Office, Washington, DC.

_____. 2008a. *Emergency Management: Observations on DHS's Preparedness for Catastrophic Disasters.* Government Accountability Office, Washington, DC.

_____. 2008b. *National Disaster Response: FEMA Should Take Action to Improve Capacity and Coordination between Government and Voluntary Sectors.* Government Accountability Office, Washington, DC.

_____. 2008c. *Homeland Security: First Responders' Ability to Detect and Model Hazardous Releases in Urban Areas Is Significantly Limited.* Government Accountability Office, Washington, DC.

_____. 2009a. *Emergency Communication: Vulnerabilities Remain and Limited Collaboration and Monitoring Hamper Federal Efforts.* Government Accountability Office, Washington, DC.

_____. 2009b. *Urban Area Security Initiative: FEMA Lacks Measures to Assess How Regional Collaboration Efforts Build Preparedness Capabilities.* Government Accountability Office, Washington, DC.

_____. 2009c. *Information Sharing: Federal Agencies Are Sharing Border and Terrorism Information with Local and Tribal Law Enforcement Agencies, but Additional Efforts Are Needed.* Government Accountability Office, Washington, DC.

_____. 2009d. *Biosurveillance: Developing a Collaboration Strategy Is Essential to Fostering Interagency Data and Resource Sharing.* Government Accountability Office, Washington, DC.

_____. 2009e. *Emergency Management: Actions to Implement Select Provisions of the Post-Katrina Emergency Management Reform Act.* Government Accountability Office, Washington, DC.

_____. 2009f. *Vulnerabilities Remain and Limited Collaboration and Monitoring Hamper Federal Efforts.* Government Accountability Office, Washington, DC.

_____. 2009g. *Emergency Communications: National Communications System Provides Programs for Priority Calling, but Planning for New Initiatives and Performance Measurement Could Be Strengthened.* Government Accountability Office, Washington, DC.

_____. 2009h. *Wildland Fire Management: Federal Agencies Have Taken Important Steps Forward, but Additional, Strategic Action Is Needed to Capitalize on Those Steps.* Government Accountability Office, Washington, DC.

_____. 2010a. *Cybersecurity: Continued Efforts Are Still Needed to Protect Infrastructure.* Government Accountability Office, Washington, DC.

_____. 2010b. *Combatting Nuclear Terrorism: Actions Needed to Better Prepare to Recover from Possible Attacks Using Radiological or Nuclear Materials.* Government Accountability Office, Washington, DC.

_____. 2010c. *Homeland Defense: Planning, Resourcing, and Training Issues Challenge DOD's Response to Domestic Chemical, Biological, Radiological, Nuclear, and High-Yield Explosive Incidents.* Government Accountability Office, Washington, DC.

_____. 2010d. *Cybersecurity: Progress Made but Challenges Remain in Defining and Coordinating the Comprehensive Initiative.* Government Accountability Office, Washington, DC.

Gomez, D., Haas, B., Ahmed, N., Tien, H., and Nathens, A. "Disaster Preparedness of Canadian Trauma Centres: The Perspective of Medical Directors of Trauma." Canadian Journal of Surgery. Journal Canadien De Chirurgie 54, No. 1 (2011): 9-16.

Gorman J.C., Cooke, N.J., and Winner, J.L. 2006. "Measuring Team Situational Awareness in Decentralized Command and Control Environments." *Ergonomics* 49 (12 and 13): 1312-1325.

"Healthcare Executives' Role in Emergency Preparedness." Healthcare Executive 25, No. 5 (2010): 104-105.

Hense, K.A., Wyler, B.D., and Kaufmann, G. "Preparedness Versus Reactiveness: An Approach to Pre-Crisis Disaster Planning." Journal of Homeland Security & Emergency Management 7, No. 1 (2010): 1-11.

Herbold, J. "Introduction to Public Health Preparedness." Texas Public Health Journal 61, No. 4 (2009): 15-21.

Hochstein, C., Arnesen, S., Goshorn, J., and Szczur, M. "Selected Resources for Emergency and Disaster Preparedness and Response from the United States National Library of Medicine." Medical Reference Services Quarterly 27, No. 1 (2008): 1-20.

Holland, J.H. *Hidden Order: How Adaptation Builds Complexity.* Reading, Massachusetts: Addison-Wesley Publishing Co, 1995, p. 55.

_____. (1995). *Hidden Order: How Adaptation Builds Complexity.* Reading, Massachusetts: Addison-Wesley Publishing Co.

Horan, J., Ritchie, L.A., Meinhold, S., Gill, D.A., Houghton, B.F., Gregg, C.E., Matheson, T., Paton, D., and Johnston, D. "Evaluating Disaster Education: The National Oceanic and Atmospheric Administration's Tsunamiready™ Community Program and Risk Awareness Education Efforts in New Hanover County, North Carolina." New Directions for Evaluation, No. 126 (2010): 79-93.

Hossain, L., and Kuti, M. "Disaster Response Preparedness Coordination through Social Networks." Disasters 34, No. 3 (2010): 755-786.

IEG World Bank. (2007). Development actions and the rising incidence of disasters. *Evaluation Brief 4.* Retrieved from: http://www.worldbank.org/ieg/docs/developing_actions.pdf

Institute of Medicine. (2006). *Emergency Medical Services at the Crossroads.* Retrieved from: http://www.iom.edu/Reports/2006/Emergecy-Medical-Services-At-the-Crossroads.aspx

International Association of Fire Chiefs, "National Fire Service Mutual Aid System Task Force," IMAS Development Plan, http://www.iafc.org/associations/4685/files/downloads/MASTF/mtlAid_IMASdevelopmentPlan.pdf (accessed February 12, 2011).

James, E. "Getting Ahead of the Next Disaster: Recent Preparedness Efforts in Indonesia." Development in Practice 18, No. 3 (2008): 424-429.

James, J.J., Subbarao, I., and Lanier, W.L. "Improving the Art and Science of Disaster Medicine and Public Health Preparedness." Mayo Clinic Proceedings. Mayo Clinic 83, No. 5 (2008): 559-562.

Joshi, A.J., and Rys, M.J. "Study on the Effect of Different Arrival Patterns on an Emergency Department's Capacity Using Discrete Event Simulation." International Journal of Industrial Engineering 18, No. 1 (2011): 40-50.

Kapucu, N. "Collaborative Emergency Management: Better Community Organizing, Better Public Preparedness and Response." Disasters 32, No. 2 (2008): 239-262.

Krajewski, M.J., Sztajnkrycer, M., and Báez, A.A. "Hospital Disaster Preparedness in the United States: New Issues, New Challenges." Internet Journal of Rescue & Disaster Medicine 4, No. 2 (2005): 32-40.

Kuhn, T.S. (1962). *The Structure of Scientific Revolutions*. Chicago & London: University of Chicago Press.

Kumar, A., Srivastava, J.P., Bhardwaj, P., and Gupta, P. "Disaster Management: A Method of Easy Survival." Internet Journal of Rescue & Disaster Medicine 8, No. 2 (2009): 1-4.

Kuntz, S.W., Frable, P., Qureshi, K., and Strong, L.L. "Association of Community Health Nursing Educators: Disaster Preparedness White Paper for Community/Public Health Nursing Educators." Public Health Nursing 25, No. 4 (2008): 362-369.

Lawson, B. (2006). *How Designers Think: The Design Process Demystified*. 4th ed. Oxford: Architectural Press.

Luck, G. "Insights on Joint Operations: The Art and Science." The Joint Warfighting Center, U.S. Joint Forces Command (September 2006), pp. 3, 12, and 22.

_____. (2006, September). "Insights on Joint Operations: The Art and Science." The Joint Warfighting Center, U.S. Joint Forces Command. (Available at https://unifiedquest.army.mil/)

Manoj, B.S., and Baker, A.H. 2007. "Communications Challenges in Emergency Response." *Communications of the ACM* 50 (3): 51-53.

Marshall County Emergency Management. *After Action Report*, December 12, 2005.

Mayer, B.W., Moss, J., and Dale, K. "Disaster and Preparedness: Lessons from Hurricane Rita." Journal of Contingencies & Crisis Management 16, No. 1 (2008): 14-23.

McAlister, V.C. "Drills and Exercises: The Way to Disaster Preparedness." Canadian Journal of Surgery. Journal Canadien De Chirurgie 54, No. 1 (2011): 7-8.

McShane, S.L., and Von Glinow, M.A. 2000. *Organizational Behavior: Emerging Realities for the Workplace Revolution*. Richard D. Irwin, Inc., New York, New York.

Miller, A. *Creation Music Festival: Chapter 1013 Special Events EMS*. Huntingdon County Emergency Management Agency, 2011.

Mishra, S., Suar, D., and Paton, D. "Is Externality a Mediator of Experience–Behavior and Information–Action Hypothesis in Disaster Preparedness?" Journal of Pacific Rim Psychology 3, No. 1 (2009): 11-19.

Montealegre, J.R., Koers, E.M., Bryson, R.S., and Murray, K.O. "An Innovative Public Health Preparedness Training Program for Graduate Students." Public Health Reports (Washington, DC: 1974) 126, No. 3 (2011): 441-446.

Morrison, A.M., and Catanzaro, A.M. "High-Fidelity Simulation and Emergency Preparedness." Public Health Nursing 27, No. 2 (2010): 164-173.

National Center for Injury Prevention and Control. "Interim Planning Guidance for Preparedness and Response to a Mass Casualty Event Resulting from Terrorist Use of Explosives." Atlanta, GA: Centers for Disease Control and Prevention, 2010

NDMS/OEP. *National Disaster Medical System*. www.ndms.dhhs.gov (Retrieved July 3, 2011).

Neustadt, R.E., and May, E.R. *Thinking In Time: The Uses of History for Decision Makers* (New York: The Free Press, 1986), pp. 34-57.

NOAA Forecast Office Paducha, KY. *Damage Survey Results for Marshall County Kentucky,* November 15, 2005.

Noll, G. "Regional Response to All-Hazards Events: A Commonwealth Perspective." Commonwealth, Vol. 15-3, May 2009.

OCMCA. *After Action Review: EMS at Woodward Dream Cruise,* November 2006.

Patterson, E.S., Roth, E.M., Woods, D.D., Chow, R., and Gomes, J.O. 2004. "Handoff Strategies in Setting with High Consequences for Failure: Lessons for Health Care Operations." *International Journal for Quality in Health Care* 16 (2): 125-132.

Poulsen K. October 23, 2007. "First Hand Reports from California Wildfires Pour Through Twitter." *Threat Level.* Accessed at http://www.wired.com/threatlevel/2007/10/firsthand-repor/ on July 30, 2010.

Ritchie, L.A., and MacDonald, W. "Enhancing Disaster and Emergency Preparedness, Response, and Recovery through Evaluation." New Directions for Evaluation, No. 126 (2010): 3-7.

Rittel, H. "On the Planning Crisis: Systems Analysis of the 'First and Second Generations.'" *Bedriftsøkonomen* 8 (1972), pp. 392-393.

Rittel, H., and Webber, M.M. "Dilemmas in a General Theory of Planning," *Policy Sciences* 4 (1973), pp. 161-167.

Rivers, F., Speraw, S., Phillips, K.D., and Lee, J. "A Review of Nurses in Disaster Preparedness and Response: Military and Civilian Collaboration." Journal of Homeland Security & Emergency Management 7, No. 1 (2010): 1-18.

Rodes, C.E., Pellizzari, E.D., Dellarco, M.J., Erickson, M.D., Vallero, D.A., Reissman, D.B., Lioy, P.J., Lippmann, M., Burke, T.A., and Goldstein, B.A. "Isea2007 Panel: Integration of Better Exposure Characterizations into Disaster Preparedness for Responders and the Public." Journal of Exposure Science & Environmental Epidemiology 18, No. 6 (2008): 541-550.

Schmitt, J.F. "A Systemic Concept for Operational Design." www.mcwl.usmc.mil/concepts/home.cfm, pp. 9-12.

Schön, D.A. *Educating the Reflective Practitioner: Toward a New Design for Teaching and Learning in the Professions* (San Francisco: Jossey-Bass Publishers, 1987), pp. 18-19 and 41-42.

Scott, L.A., Carson, D.S., and Greenwell, I.B. "Disaster 101: A Novel Approach to Disaster Medicine Training for Health Professionals." Journal of Emergency Medicine 39, No. 2 (2010): 220-226.

Seale, G.S. "Emergency Preparedness as a Continuous Improvement Cycle: Perspectives from a Postacute Rehabilitation Facility." Rehabilitation Psychology 55, No. 3 (2010): 247-254.

Serino, R., *Medical Consequence Management Plan for the 2004 Democratic National Convention,* LLIS.gov, 2011.

Shear, W.B. "Small Business Administration: Additional Steps Needed to Enhance Agency Preparedness for Future Disasters: Gao-07-114." GAO Reports, (2007): 1.

"Small Business Administration: Response to the Gulf Coast Hurricanes Highlights Need for Enhanced Disaster Preparedness: Gao-07-484t." GAO Reports, (2007): 1.

Sorrells, W.T., Downing, G.R., Blakesley, P., Pendall, D.W., Walk, J.K., and Wallwork, R.D. (2005). *Systemic Operational Design: An Introduction.* School of Advanced Military Studies, U.S. Army Command and General Staff College. (Available at http://www-cgsc.army.mil/carl/contentdm/home.htm)

South Central Task Force. *Lebanon (PA) Veterans Administration Medical Center Evacuation-EMS Operations After Action Report/Improvement Plan*, November 2010.

Staudenherz, A., and Leitha, T. "Medical Preparedness in Radiation Accidents: A Matter of Logistics and Communication Not Treatment!" International Journal of Occupational & Environmental Medicine 2, No. 3 (2011): 133-142.

Strange, J. (2002). *Centers of Gravity and Critical Vulnerabilities: Building on the Clausewitzian Foundation So That We Can All Speak the Same Language.* 2nd ed. Quantico, Virginia: Marine Corps University.

Swienton, R.E., Subbarao, I., and Coule, P.L. "Healthcare Disasters: Local Preparedness, Global Response!" Strengthening National Public Health Preparedness and Response to Chemical, Biological and Radiological Agent Threats 20, No. 1 (2007): 11-14.

Thomas K., Hallock, K., and Bergethon, P.R. 2008. "The Need for Cross Discipline Awareness and Interoperability in the First Responder and Emergency Management Communities." In proceedings of *The Cornwallis Group XIII: Analysis of Societal Conflict and Counter Insurgency.* Cornwallis Park, Nova Scotia, Canada.

Top, M., Gider, O., and Tas, Y. "An Investigation of Hospital Disaster Preparedness in Turkey." Journal of Homeland Security & Emergency Management 7, No. 1 (2010): 1-19.

Utah Department of Public Health. *Ford Ironman St. George Triathlon,* May 2010.

van Wyk, E., Bean, W.L., and Yadavalli, V.S.S. "Modeling of Uncertainty in Minimizing the Cost of Inventory for Disaster Relief." South African Journal of Industrial Engineering 22, No. 1 (2011): 1-11.

Walker, D.M. "Hurricane Katrina: Gao's Preliminary Observations Regarding Preparedness, Response, and Recovery: Gao-06-442t." GAO Reports, (2006): 1.

Woodbury, G.L. "Washington State Hazard Identification and Vulnerability Assessment." Washington Emergency Management Division, (2005): 16-24.

This page was intentionally left blank.

www.ingramcontent.com/pod-product-compliance
Lightning Source LLC
Chambersburg PA
CBHW081616170426
43195CB00041B/2856